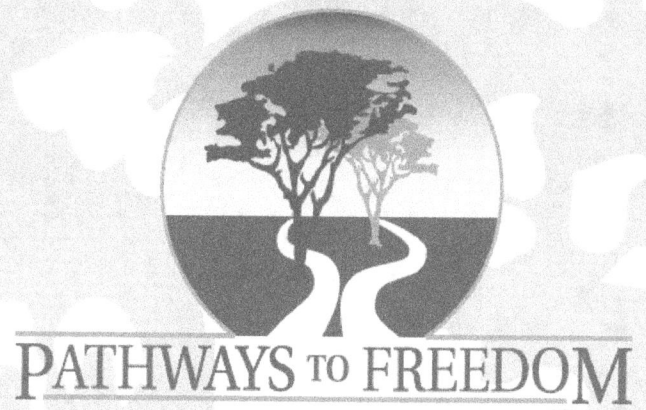

PATHWAYS TO FREEDOM

WINNING THE FIGHT AGAINST TOBACCO

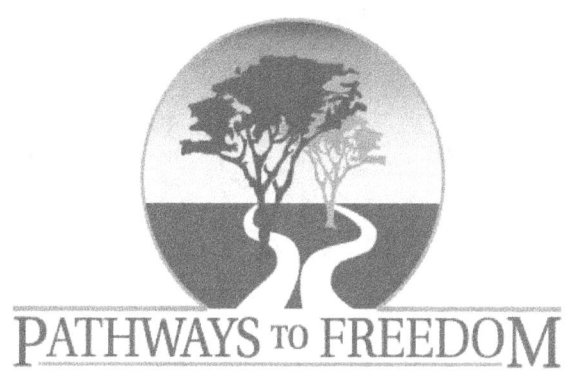

PATHWAYS TO FREEDOM

WINNING THE FIGHT AGAINST TOBACCO

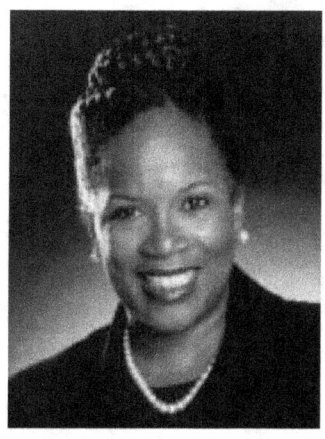

Lucille C. Perez, M.D.
102nd President
National Medical Association

"The National Medical Association (NMA) supports the distribution of *Pathways to Freedom* to the African American community. Tobacco use is a major cause of death and disease for Black people. *Pathways to Freedom* has been a tremendous blessing for Black smokers, their families and friends, and the greater community. The NMA endorses *Pathways to Freedom* and urges all persons concerned with the well-being of Black people to use these materials, support their distribution, and make them part of all health programs and services intended for the African American community."

Authors
Robert G. Robinson, Dr.P.H.
Charyn D. Sutton, B.A.
Denise A. James, B.S., M.Ed., CHES
Carole Tracy Orleans, Ph.D.

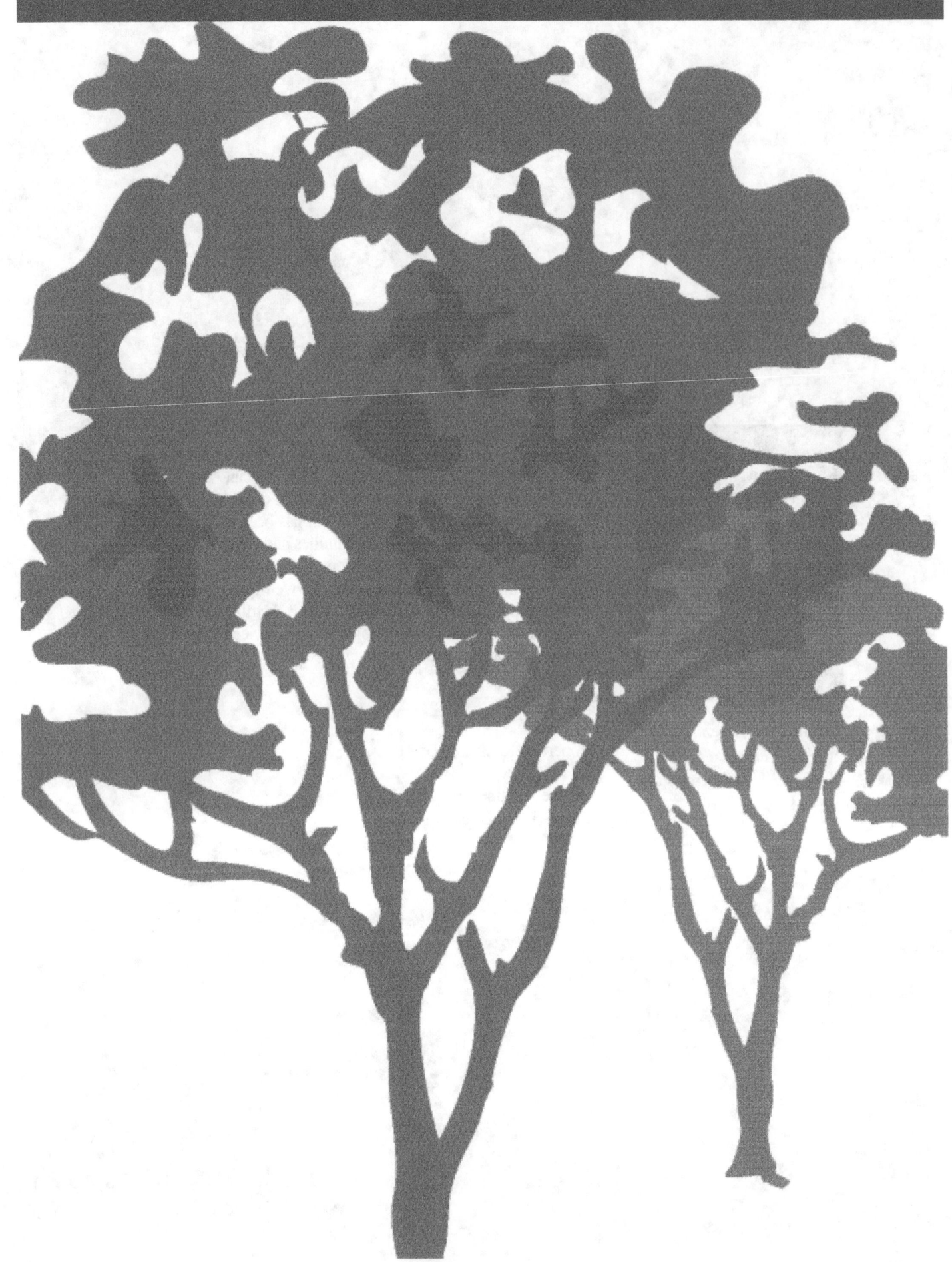

Pathways to Freedom

The freedom we are talking about is freedom from tobacco. Freeing ourselves from the need for cigarettes is a step on the path to taking more control over our lives. The *Pathways to Freedom* guide is one answer to the major problem of smoking for Blacks in America. For smokers, it provides a place to start. It helps friends and families be part of the solution and provides strategies for community members who want to educate people about the dangers of tobacco. This is your guide. It was put together with the help of Black churches, tenant groups, the Prince Hall Shriners, Daughters of Isis, and other members of the community.

The Guide Has Three Parts

- **Education**—Informs you of how tobacco use affects the Black community.

- **How to Quit**—Tells you and those around you how you can quit smoking.

- **Community Organization**—Shows you how communities can work together to fight against the tobacco industry.

Freeing ourselves from the need for a drug like nicotine in cigarettes is a step on the path to taking more control over our lives.

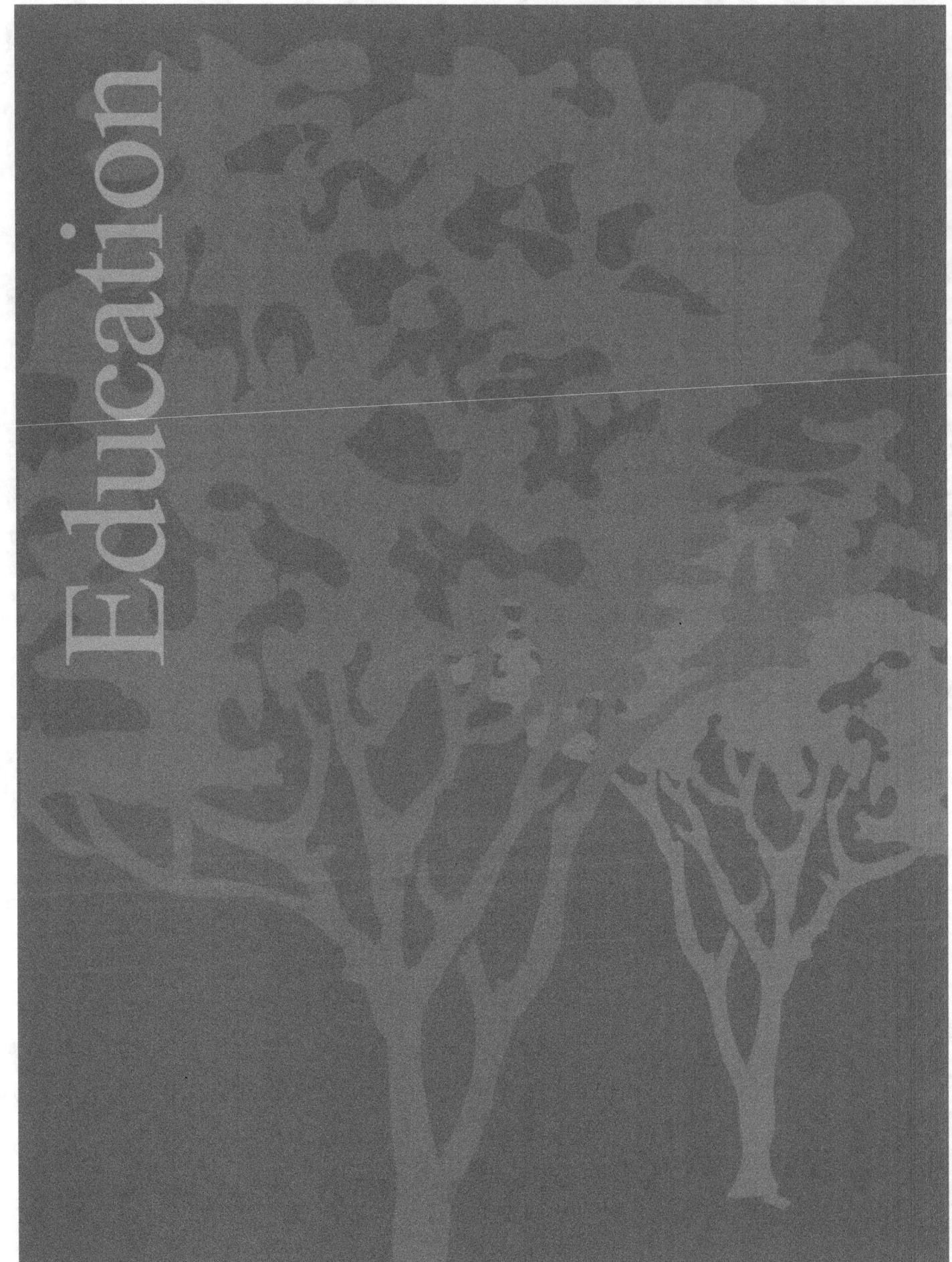

Education

Meet the Freeman Family

Finding the path that takes us away from tobacco isn't easy. No one way works for everybody. That is why we asked the Freeman family to help.

The Freeman family lives in Anytown, USA. The family has a father, a mother, and three children. The grandparents and Aunt Noreen (the father's sister and mother's best friend) are also part of the family. Granddaddy's great-grandfather took the last name "Freeman" in the mid-1800s when slavery ended. ▮

The Freemans are a lot like many Black people you know. Some of them are smokers, and some are not.

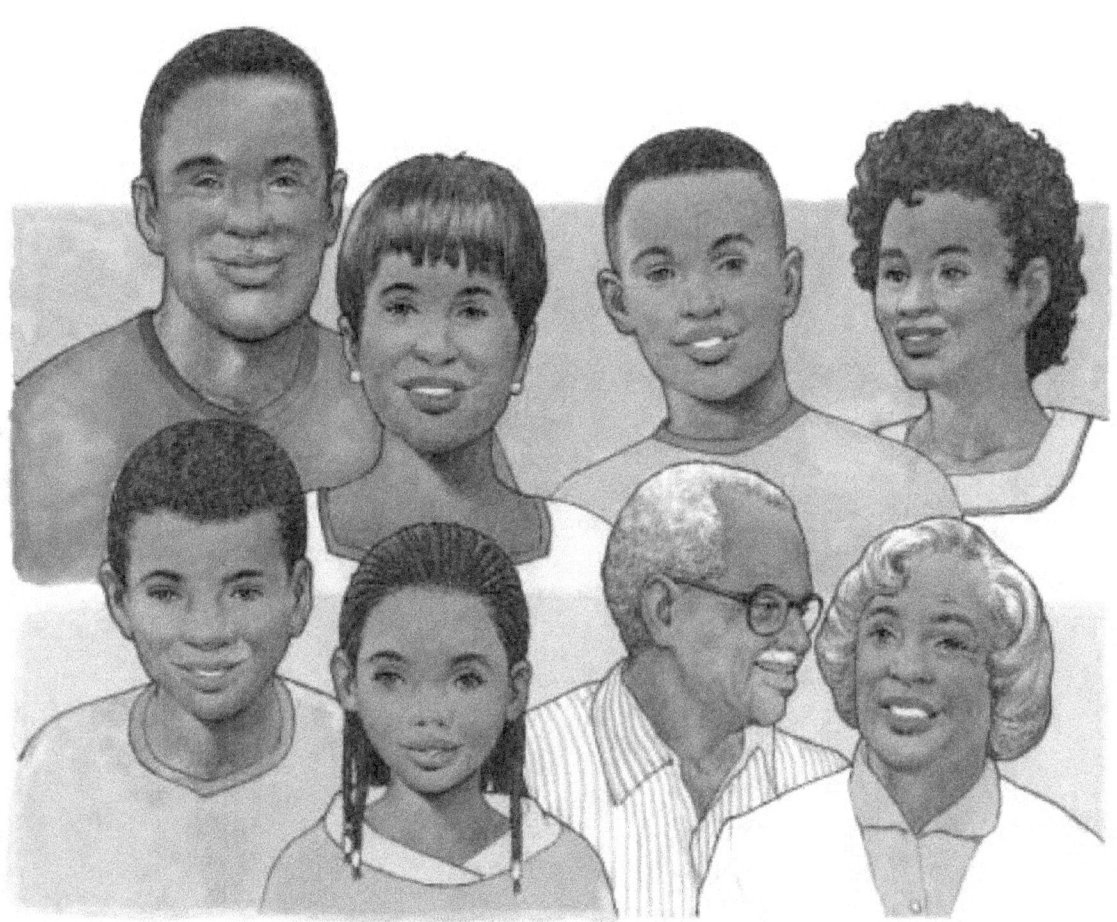

The Freeman family...Top row, from the left: father Sam, mother Dot, older son Tyrone, and Aunt Noreen (father's sister and mother's best friend). Bottom row, from the left: younger son M.J., daughter Nia, Granddaddy, and Grandma. Granddaddy, father Sam, and Aunt Noreen are smokers.

What Smoking Cigarettes Does to Us

"He who conceals his disease cannot expect to be cured."

– Ethiopian proverb

Smoking causes 1 out of every 5 deaths in the United States. The average smoker dies 7–8 years too early. Smokers are also more likely to get diseases that make it hard to lead an active life.

Before the 1950s, smoking was far less common among Blacks than Whites. This is not true anymore. There are now more than 8 million African Americans who smoke. Because more Blacks are smoking, deaths of Black people who smoke have gone way up.

Each year, more than 47,000 Black people in the United States die from diseases they get just because they smoke. That includes African Americans and also Black people who have come to the United States from other parts of the world. Tobacco-related diseases kill more Black Americans each year than car crashes, AIDS, murders, and drug and alcohol abuse put together.

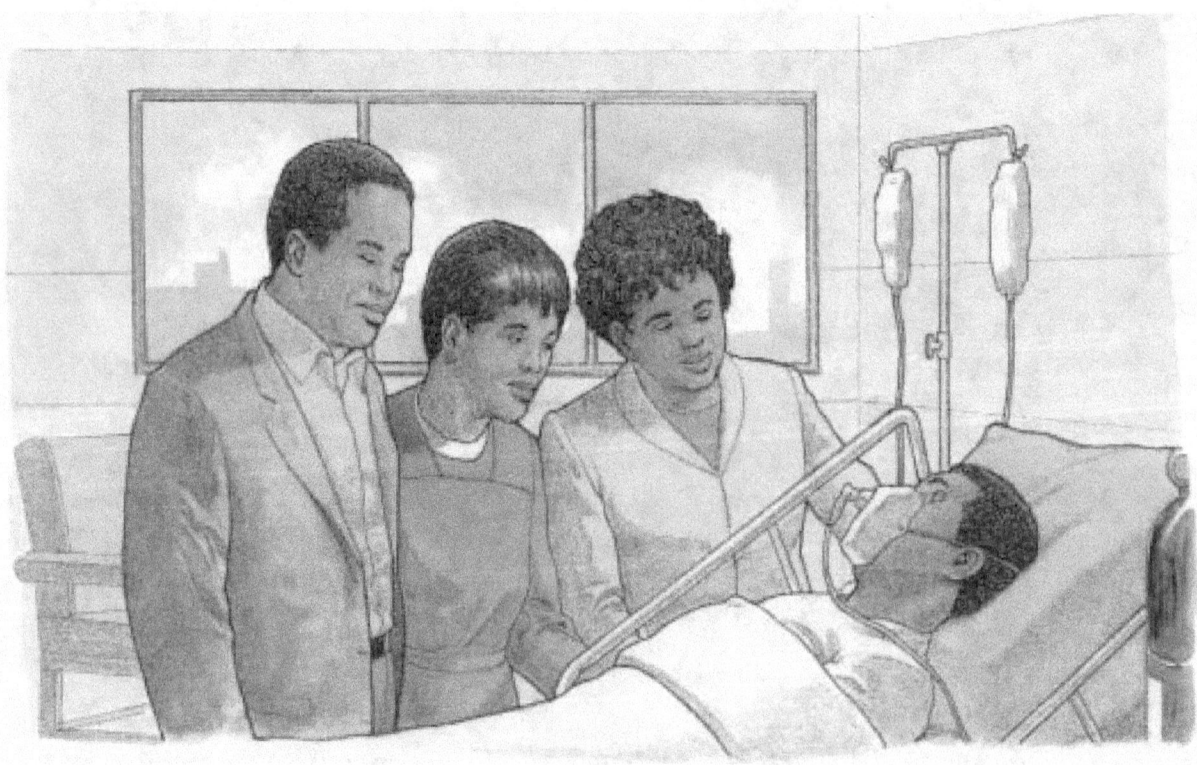

Sickness caused by smoking puts people in the hospital every day.

Some Other Problems That Come From Smoking

Smoking even a few cigarettes a day does damage. Cigarettes are a major cause of heart attacks, and they can also damage the blood vessels. Smoking can lead to strokes and emphysema. **Smoking can cause cancers of the lungs, throat, mouth, bladder, cervix, stomach, and kidney.**

Women face special risks from smoking. More Black women today get lung cancer than get breast cancer. Smoking causes problems during pregnancy. A baby that is born to a smoker may be sickly or even die. Black men are 50% more likely to get lung cancer than White men.

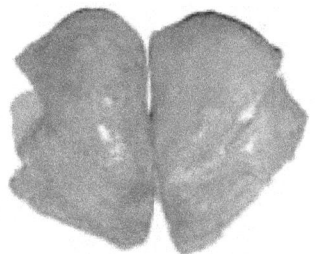

Baby's Healthy Lungs

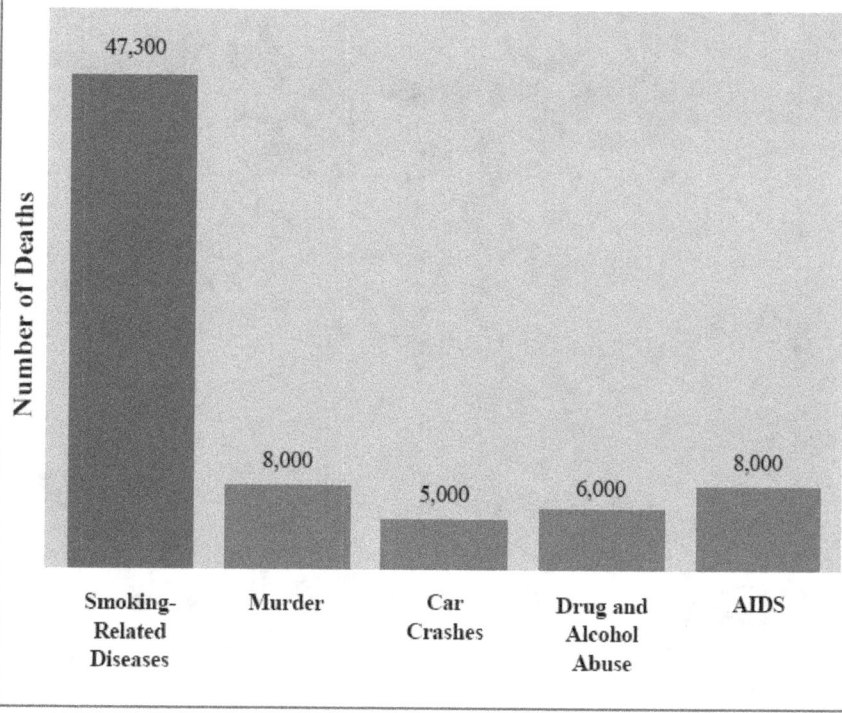

Leading Causes of Death for African Americans

Each year, more Black Americans die from diseases caused by smoking than from murders, AIDS, drug and alcohol abuse, and car crashes put together.

Number of Deaths

47,300

8,000

5,000

6,000

8,000

Smoking-Related Diseases   Murder   Car Crashes   Drug and Alcohol Abuse   AIDS

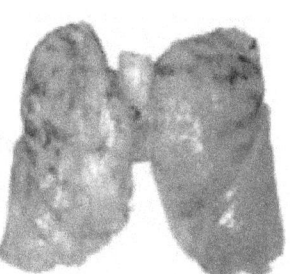

Mildly Diseased Adult Lungs

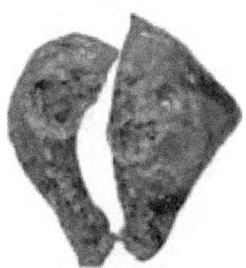

Severely Diseased Adult Lungs

Breathing Someone Else's Smoke

> "Nothing can
> be changed
> until it is
> faced."
>
> – *James Baldwin*

Secondhand smoke is the smoke that is exhaled or that comes from the burning end of a cigarette, pipe, or cigar. Secondhand smoke can come in through cracks in the walls. It can hang around in hallways and doorways where people have been smoking.

Breathing someone else's smoke can be deadly, especially if you live or work in a place where people smoke. That is why it is so important for smokers to go all the way outside if they want a cigarette. When one person smokes inside, it can cause problems for everyone else.

Children who are around tobacco smoke in their homes have more health problems like asthma and ear infections. They are sicker and stay in bed more. They miss more school days than children whose homes are smoke-free. Babies who live in homes with secondhand smoke are more likely to die as infants than other babies.

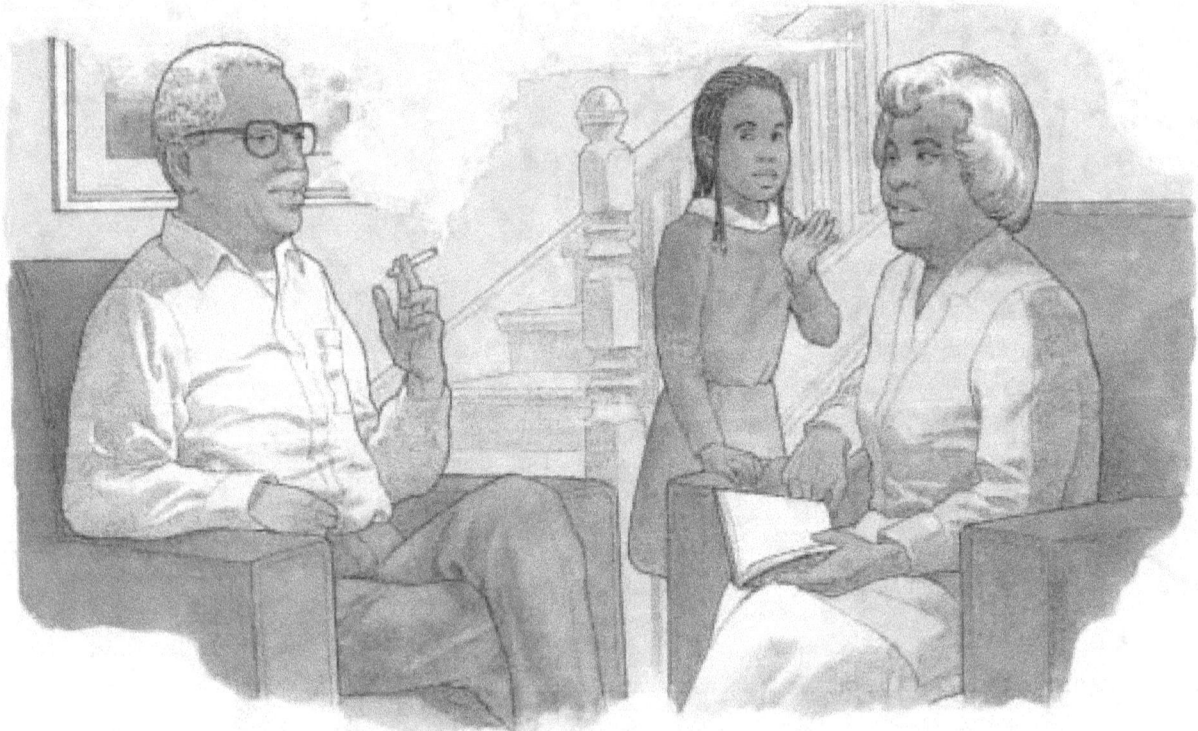

Grandma to Granddaddy: "I wish you wouldn't smoke those cigarettes around your granddaughter Nia. It's hard for her to breathe with all that smoke."

Smoke Hurts Those Around You

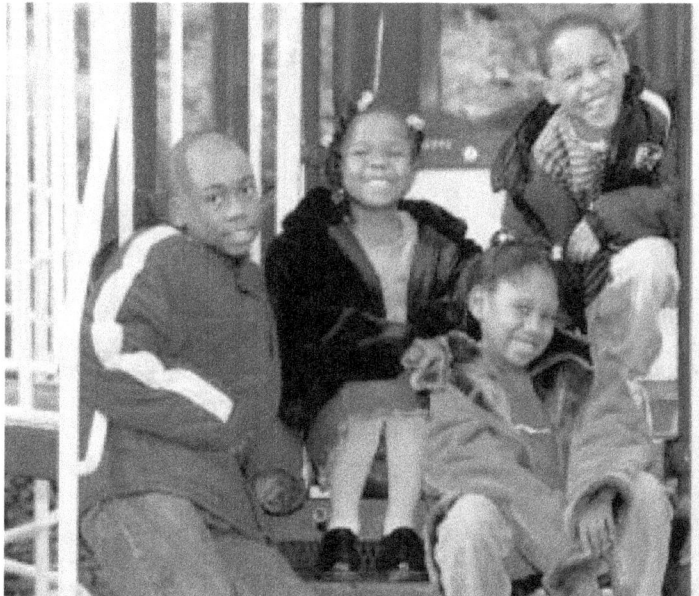

"We are happier when the people we love don't smoke."

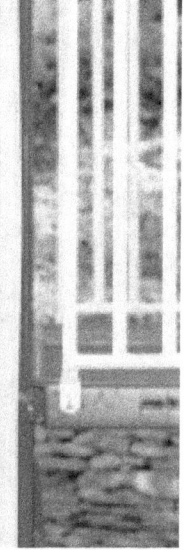

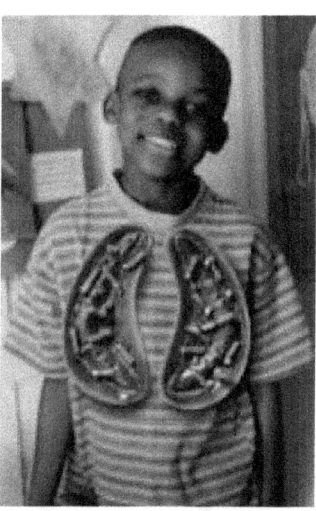

If you smoke around your child, he inhales many of the same poisons that you do.

The number of Black children with asthma is 25% higher than the number of White children with asthma. These children can have attacks if they breathe cigarette smoke. African American adults are 2 to 3 times more likely than White adults to go to the hospital if they have an asthma attack.

In many Black communities, people don't say much about secondhand smoke. They don't want to hurt a smoker's feelings. It is often hard for younger Black people to say anything at all. To speak out would seem rude and disrespectful.

Most smokers know that it is important for them to quit for their own health. What smokers need to understand is that their secondhand smoke can make people around them sick too. It can take as long as 2 weeks for the nicotine in tobacco smoke to clear out from a room where people have been smoking.

Tobacco Products: They Sell, We Buy

"All actions are

judge by the

motive

prompting them."

– From the sayings of Muhammed (Hadith)

Tobacco companies sell billions of cigarettes and cigars in Black communities. One reason is because of target marketing. That's when a company picks out certain groups and uses ads to get their attention. Cigarette companies use target marketing all the time—not only to the Black community, but also to other groups like women, gays and lesbians, and blue-collar workers.

A report by the tobacco company says it is the money: **"Clearly, the sole reason for interest in ... black ... communities is the actual and potential sales of ... products within these communities ...."** (Brown and Williamson Tobacco Corporation).

NO community should ever be targeted with a product that kills.

Tobacco companies reach the Black community with glitzy ads that give the wrong message—especially to children. Tobacco ads show only beautiful people. They never show people who become sick and die because they smoked.

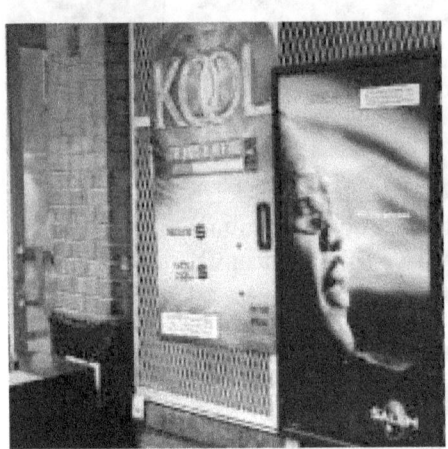 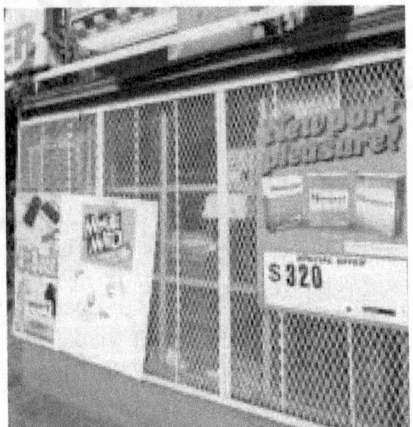
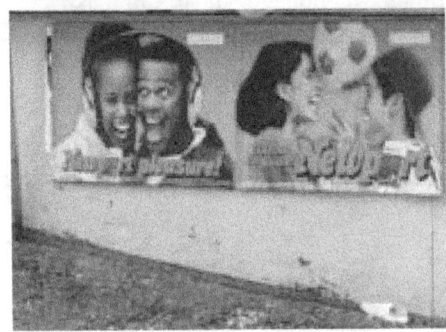 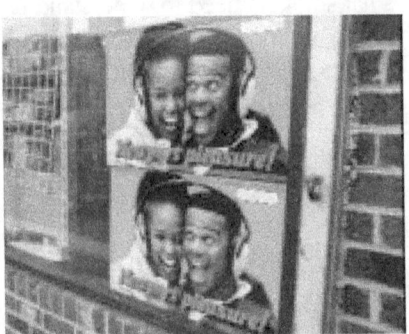

It is hard to miss all the cigarette ads in the community.

False Friends

Over the years, tobacco companies have given money to support Black music, sports, theater, dance programs, and art shows. But the money that they give away is much less than the money they make from selling cigarettes to Black people. **In fact, the money that African American smokers spend on cigarettes in a single day could send more than 2,500 Black students to college for an entire year.**

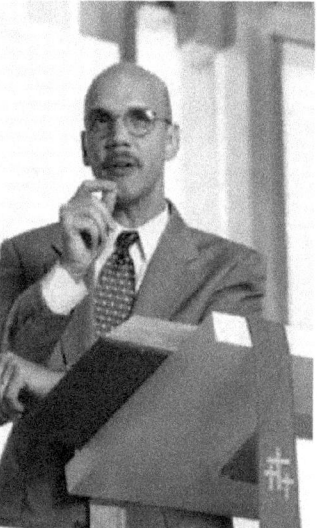

Your Cigarette Money Could Buy...

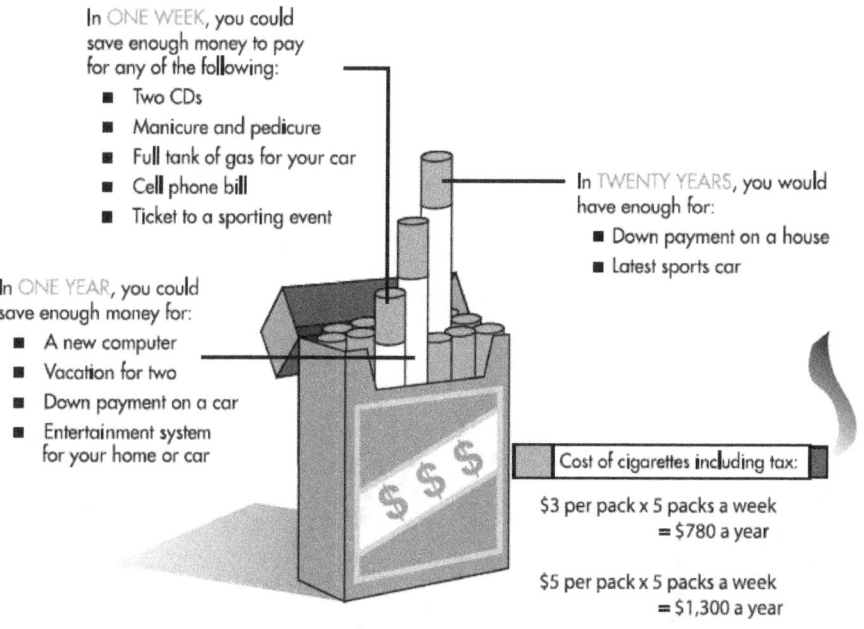

In ONE WEEK, you could save enough money to pay for any of the following:
- Two CDs
- Manicure and pedicure
- Full tank of gas for your car
- Cell phone bill
- Ticket to a sporting event

In ONE YEAR, you could save enough money for:
- A new computer
- Vacation for two
- Down payment on a car
- Entertainment system for your home or car

In TWENTY YEARS, you would have enough for:
- Down payment on a house
- Latest sports car

Cost of cigarettes including tax:

$3 per pack x 5 packs a week = $780 a year

$5 per pack x 5 packs a week = $1,300 a year

$7 per pack x 5 packs a week = $1,820 a year

"If we just count the number of people it kills, tobacco is the number one health problem facing the Black community."

Why Do Smokers Keep Smoking?

"My people
are destroyed
for lack of
knowledge."

*– Old Testament, KJV,
Hosea 4:6*

Some people think that smoking is just a bad habit. But smoking is more than a habit. Most smokers' bodies need the nicotine in cigarettes or they go into withdrawal. Needing something that much is called addiction. That's why most smokers keep smoking even when the cigarette prices go up. That's why a smoker will go outside to smoke even if the weather is raining, cold, or blazing hot.

Most smokers are addicted. If a person reaches for a cigarette within 30 minutes after waking up, that tells the tale. According to the U.S. Surgeon General, the nicotine in cigarettes can be as addictive as cocaine or heroin.

Many people say they smoke cigarettes to unwind and to feel more relaxed. But studies show that smoking actually raises a person's blood pressure and heart rate.

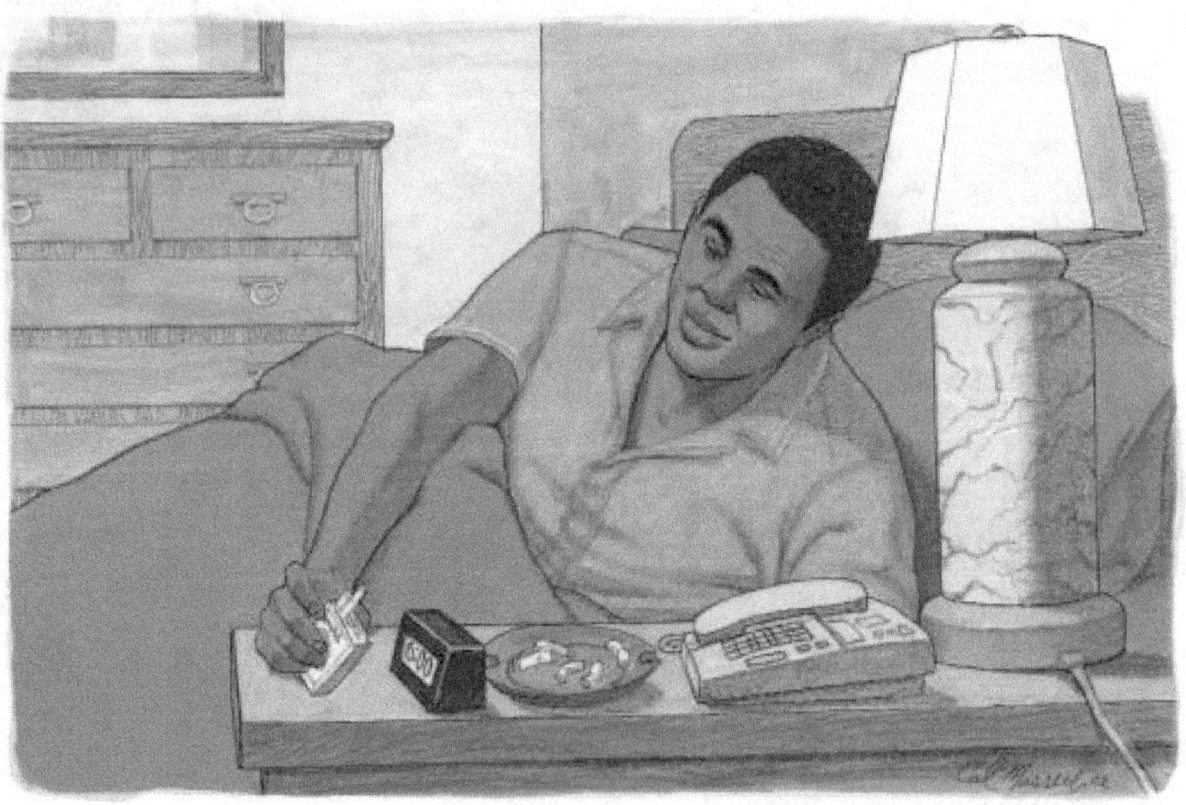

You know you are hooked when you reach for a cigarette first thing in the morning.

What's Keeping You from Quitting?

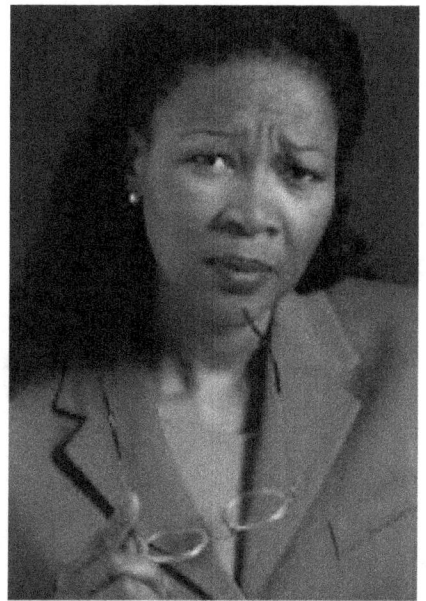

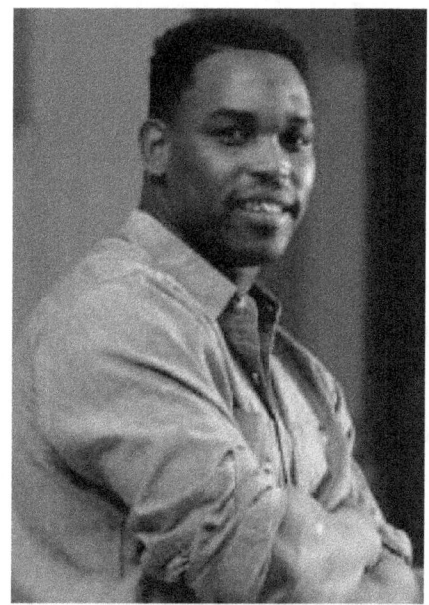

"I want to quit, but the pressure at work really gets to me. Then there is the addiction. Sometimes I just crave a cigarette."

"I used to think that cigarettes helped me cope. But the way I see it now, they just add to my problems."

The Dangers of Menthol

Menthol cigarette brands have been the top sellers among African American smokers for many years. In fact, 3 out of 4 Black smokers buy menthols. Chemicals are added to menthol cigarettes to give them a fresh, minty taste. This can make it easier for a smoker to inhale deeply, which may allow more chemicals to enter the lungs.

Menthol in cigarettes does not make smoking safer. In fact, menthol may even make things worse. No one knows for sure. What we do know is that the only safe number of cigarettes to smoke is zero.

What's in Cigarette Smoke?

There are 4,700 chemicals in cigarette smoke, and at least 60 are known to cause cancer in humans. Some of the chemicals in cigarette smoke are:

Acetone–fingernail polish remover

Ammonia–toilet cleaner

Arsenic–rat poison

Butane–cigarette lighter fluid

Cadmium–used in paint

Carbon Monoxide–car exhaust fumes

Formaldehyde–used to preserve dead people

Hexamine–barbecue lighter

Hydrogen Cyanide–gas chamber poison

Methanol–rocket fuel

Naphthalene–mothballs

Nicotine–insecticide/addictive drug

Nitrobenzene–gasoline additive

Stearic Acid–candle wax

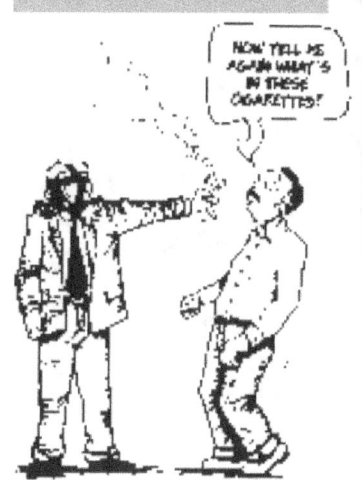

How to Quit

Where Are You in Your Plans to Quit?

I'm not ready to quit smoking.
Read this guide for reasons why you should quit.

I'll be ready to quit smoking soon.
Don't wait too long. This guide will give you ideas on how to get ready to quit.

I'm ready to quit right now.
Great! Read on for ideas that can help you to quit and stay quit.

I used to smoke, but I've quit.
Great! This guide can help you to stay quit.

I quit before, but I'm smoking again.
This guide is for you, too. People quitting cigarettes often try many times before they succeed. Read on for tips to help you to quit for good.

A few people can stop smoking just by throwing away their cigarettes. But for most people, quitting smoking is not that easy. Quitting takes more than willpower. It takes a solid plan.

Pathways to Freedom is a quit-smoking plan that has worked for many African Americans. It looks at ways to end the smoking addiction. This guide tells about choosing a Quit Day. You will learn about medicines and counseling to help you quit. There is advice on handling stress, fighting off the urge to smoke, and keeping extra pounds away.

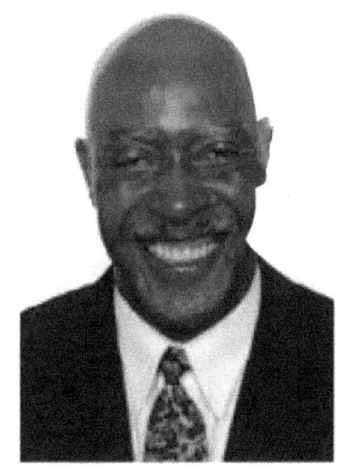

"I set a goal of quitting by my birthday. To get ready, I used the plan in the *Pathways to Freedom* guide and I did it."

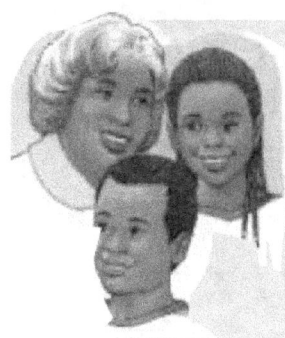

And If You Don't Smoke . . .

This guide is for you, too. Just look for advice from Nia, Grandma, and M.J. You'll find ideas and hints to help people you love who are trying to quit smoking. Smokers with support from family and friends are more successful in quitting smoking.

Fight the Smoking Triggers: You Can Quit!

"Little by little the bird builds its nest."

– Haitian proverb

Most smokers like to smoke at special times. It may be right after a meal or when they are at a party with friends. Some people light up whenever they talk on the phone or get into a car. Other triggers for smoking can be watching television, playing cards, or reading a book. Drinking alcohol or a cup of coffee can make a person want a cigarette.

Often the triggers for smoking are feelings. Smokers sometimes smoke more when they are upset, bothered, or stressed out. Lighting up is a way of shutting down. It is a way of coping with problems—like losing a job, breaking up with a loved one, or having someone crash into your car.

Nicotine is an addiction, but quitting is possible. There are many ways a smoker can gain control over urges to smoke. Here are some ideas.

Make a list of the times when you always reach for a cigarette. Pick one of those times. Then, do something else instead of smoking. For example, let's say you always smoke when you are on the phone. Put some paper and color pens by the phone instead of cigarettes. To keep from being tempted, remove the ashtrays and matches from the telephone stand. When you're on the telephone, try doodling instead of puffing.

Alcohol can act as a trigger for smoking. While you are quitting smoking, try not to drink liquor, beer, or wine for 3 months.

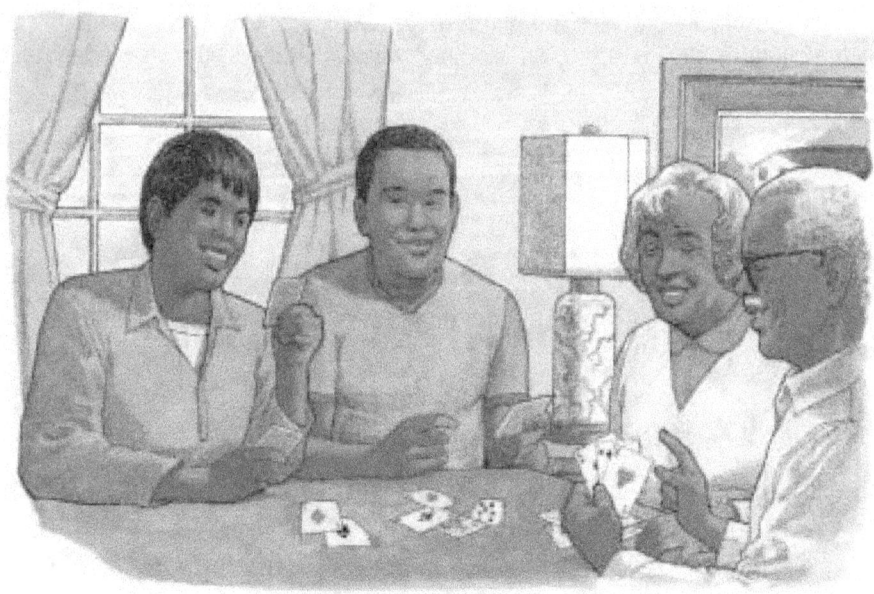

Sam: "I usually smoke when I play cards. I'm trying to break that habit."

Things to Do Instead of Smoking

If you always smoke in the car, take away the lighter. Put your cigarettes in the trunk while you are driving. Instead of smoking, listen to some soft music.

Don't try to do everything at once. Change one thing at a time. Stop smoking at one special time. It may not be easy, but stick to it until you succeed! Don't give in. Then go on to the next thing you want to change.

Keep going until you have checked off all the smoking triggers on your list. If you can stop smoking at your favorite times, you are well on your way to stopping all the time. These quit ideas are useful for the light smoker as well as for the heavy tobacco user.

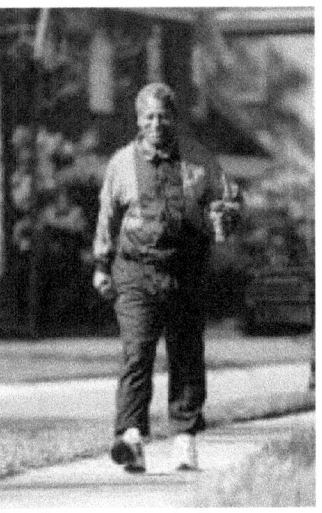

"Exercising is part of my life now. I try to work out almost every day."

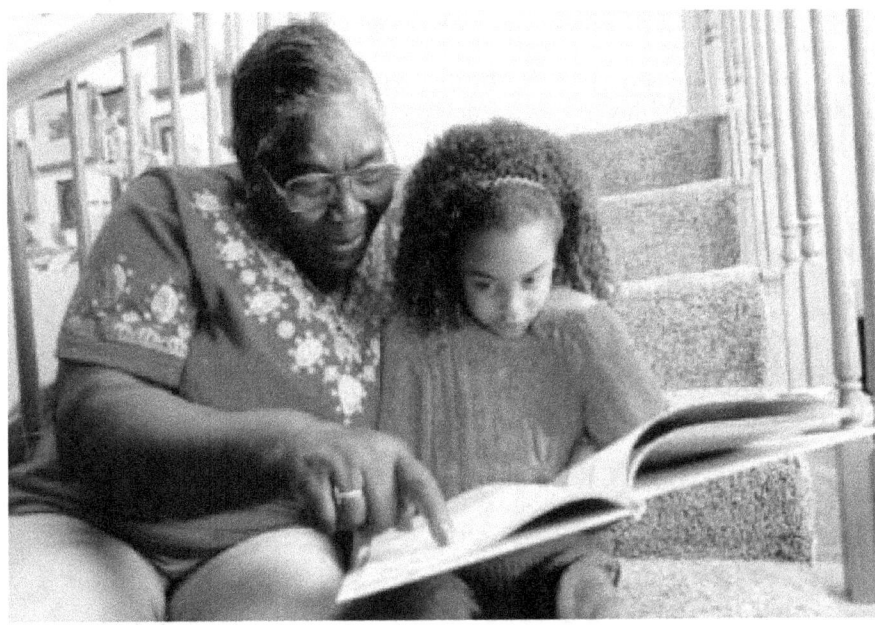

"Now that I've stopped smoking, I feel I can be a much better role model for my granddaughter. That really makes me feel good."

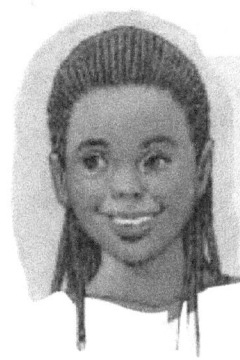

If You Want to Help

"Don't ask to go places where people will be smoking. Suggest a movie or a smoke-free restaurant instead."

Ending the Tobacco Addiction

"We must
learn to respect
ourselves."

– Audre Lorde

Why do most smokers have trouble quitting? It is because they are addicted to the nicotine in their cigarettes.

Smoking cigarettes gives a smoker regular jolts of nicotine. After a while, the body gets used to it. For an addicted smoker, being without nicotine brings on feelings of withdrawal.

But the nicotine is NOT what causes the major health risks of smoking. Cigarettes are filled with thousands of other chemicals. Doctors believe the deadly chemicals in cigarettes and tobacco smoke cause the bad health effects of smoking. For example, most brands that Blacks smoke are high in tar. Tar in cigarettes causes lung cancer. Cigarettes also have carbon monoxide, which takes oxygen from the blood and can lead to strokes.

Studies show that Black smokers actually want to quit more than most other groups. Hundreds of thousands of Black smokers have quit smoking already. More try and succeed every day. So can you.

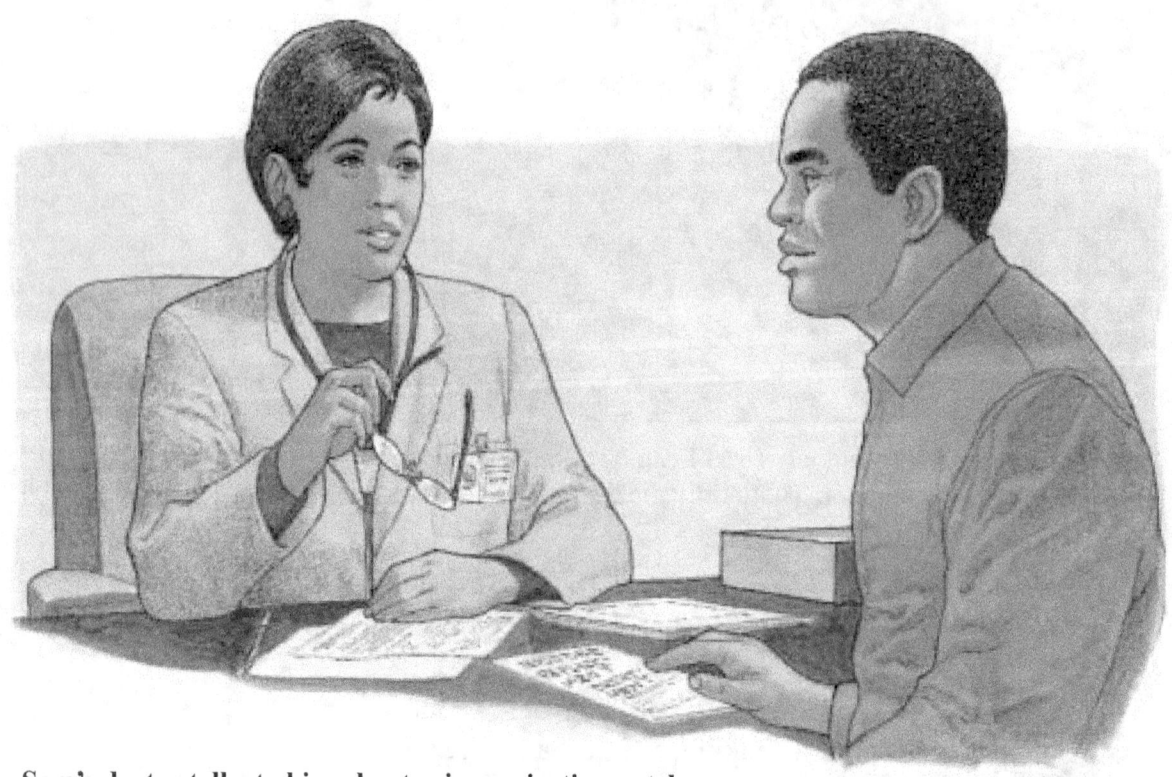

Sam's doctor talks to him about using a nicotine patch.

Ways to Fight Nicotine Addiction

Using products that replace the nicotine in cigarettes and cigars for a short time can greatly increase the chances of a smoker quitting. These products have small amounts of nicotine without all the other chemicals. The nicotine products come as patches, gum, lozenges, inhalers, and sprays. The idea is to help the body get over its need for nicotine—little by little.

There are also pills to help smokers quit. A smoker usually begins taking the pills a week or two before the Quit Day. They also reduce feelings of not having nicotine. However, they do not have nicotine in them. The first nicotine-free quit-smoking pill—Zyban®—was approved for use in the United States in 1997. Other products are in the planning stage.

Medicines that help smokers quit can be bought over-the-counter and by prescription. Your doctor or pharmacist may be helpful in figuring out which medicine is best for you. ▪

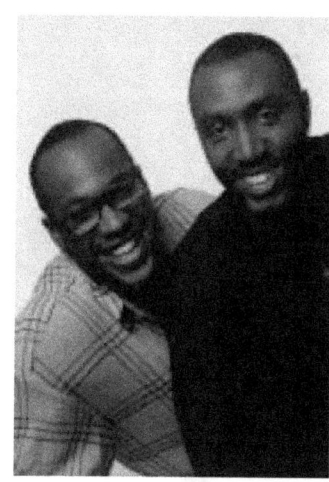

"Patience and strong support from my friend helped me quit. He really understood what I was up against."

Quit Smoking Medicines Work Best With:

▪ Help from your doctor

▪ One-on-one counseling

▪ Call-in telephone quitlines

▪ Quit smoking classes or support groups

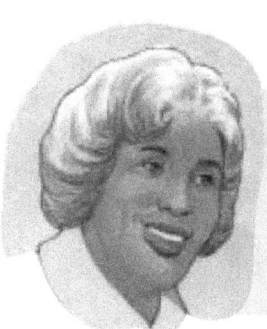

If You Want to Help

"People can get very edgy when they are trying to quit smoking. Be understanding. Their grumpiness will pass with time."

Set a Quit Day: Take the First Step

"Take the first step in faith."

– Dr. Martin Luther King, Jr.

Doctors say you should choose a specific Quit Day. Having a Quit Day gives you a goal to reach. It is a promise to keep to yourself and your loved ones. Setting a Quit Day 2 to 3 weeks in advance gives you time to get ready.

There is no "perfect" time to quit. But some times are better than others. It is much harder to quit when you face a family crisis or a big problem at work. Pick a time when things are going well. You may pick a day that is celebrated by the community, such as Dr. Martin Luther King, Jr., Day.

Circle your Quit Day on the calendar. Write it down. Carry it with you. Tell your family and friends. Share the *Pathways to Freedom* guide with them so they can help you succeed. Check to see if your doctor can tell you about any medicines that can help you quit.

If you know people who used to smoke, ask them how they quit. If you live or work with other smokers, ask them not to offer you a cigarette, even if you ask. And don't be surprised if a friend or family member wants to quit smoking along with you.

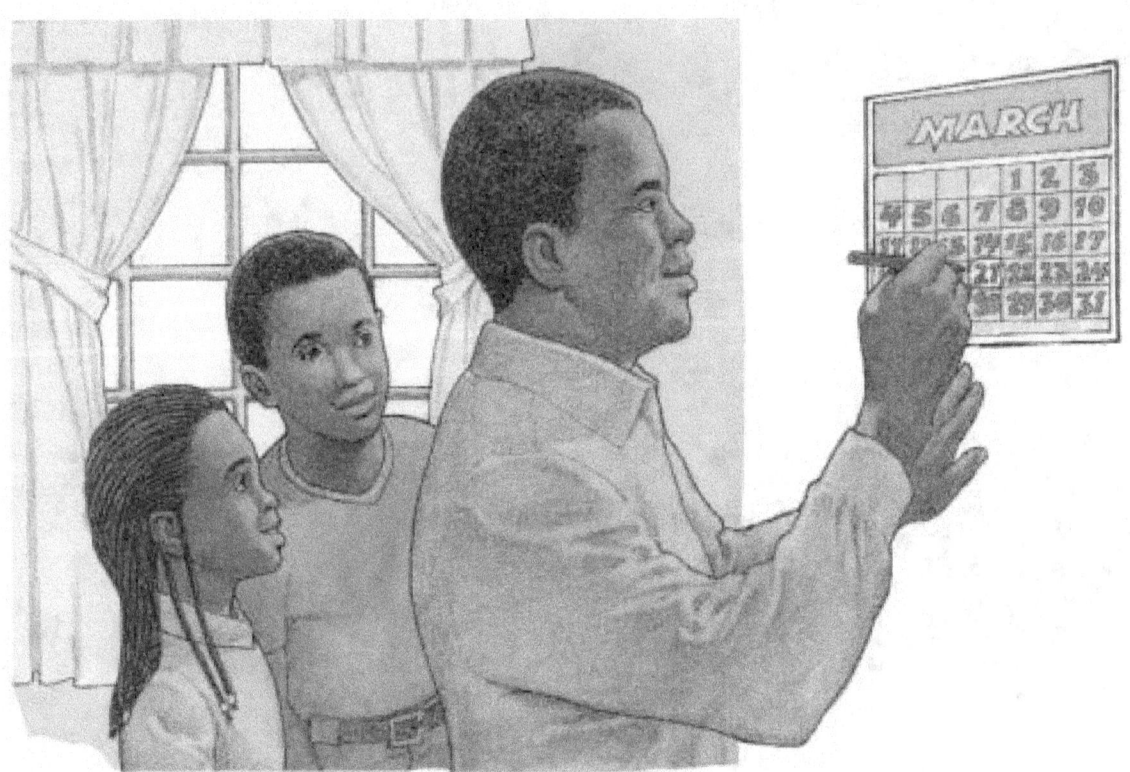

Sam: "I'm ready to quit. Setting a Quit Day is my first step."

It Can Be Done

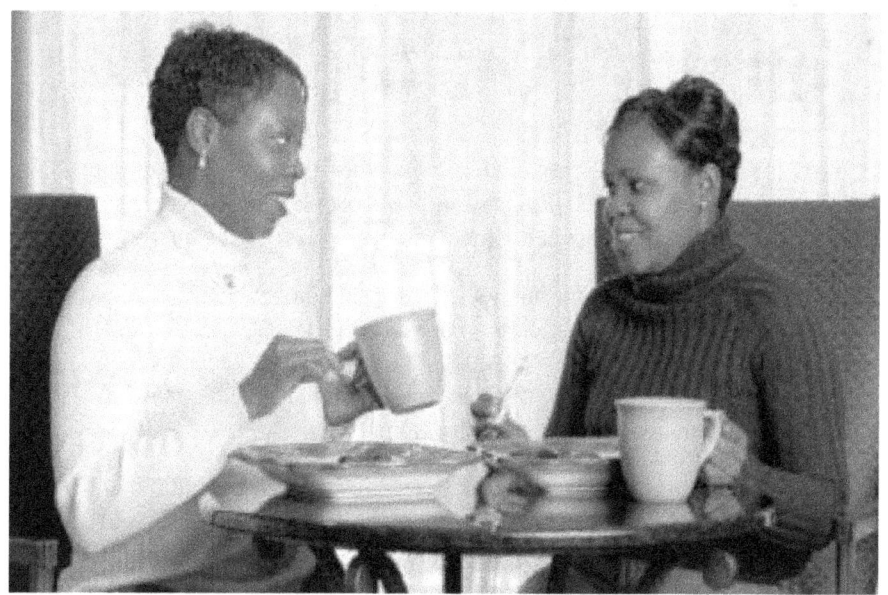

"My best friend and I picked the same Quit Day. That way, there were two of us going through the tough times together."

Your Quit Day is very important. Ask anyone you know who used to smoke. Twenty years from now, the day you gave up cigarettes for good will be a day that you remember.

Think positive thoughts. Say to yourself, "I can do it this time!" even if you have tried before. Think about how much better you will feel after you quit for good.

The Night Before

- Throw out all your cigarettes, every last one! Get them out of hiding places, like pockets, handbags, and glove compartments.

- Get rid of lighters, matches, and ashtrays. Make sure there is nothing around that reminds you of cigarettes.

- If you plan to use medicines to help you quit, make sure you know how to use them. Ask your doctor or pharmacist if you have questions.

- Stock up on sugar-free gum and mints, carrots, celery, or cloves, so you always have something to reach for instead of a cigarette.

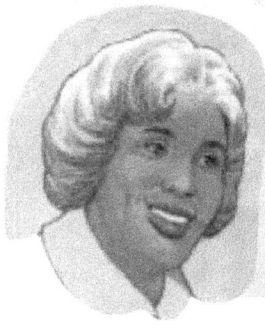

If You Want to Help

"If you have a friend who's trying to quit, be there for them. They need someone to tell them it's going to be all right."

Don't Get Side-tracked: You Are Not Alone

"Make no promise for tomorrow if you are able to keep it today."

– Iyanla Vanzant

One of the problems some smokers face when they try to quit is that other people around them are still smoking. They see people with cigarettes everywhere they look—on street corners, on posters, on TV, in movies.

That can make quitting harder but not impossible. Smokers don't have to battle smoking on their own. Quit-smoking materials, medicines, and program information are given out by doctors, local hospitals, health care centers, churches, and community organizations. Some are free, some are low cost, and some can be purchased without a prescription.

Some people use prayer as part of their personal approach to quitting. Others chant or think quiet thoughts. Faith communities often sponsor quit-smoking classes and call-in prayer lines. Some hold special Smoke-free Sabbath services to help smokers quit. Drawing on spiritual support and a person's belief in God or a "higher power" can lessen the stress of quitting smoking.

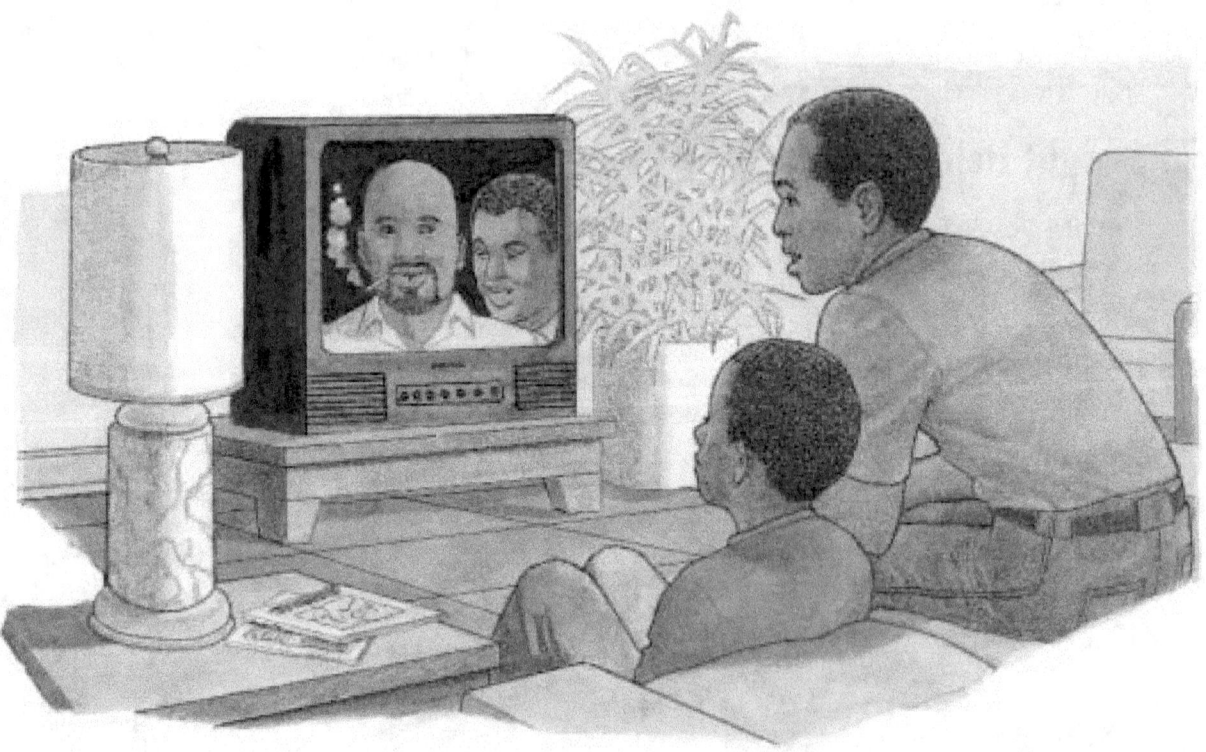

Smoking can look great when celebrities do it, but it isn't so great in real life.

Quit Smoking Programs Can Help

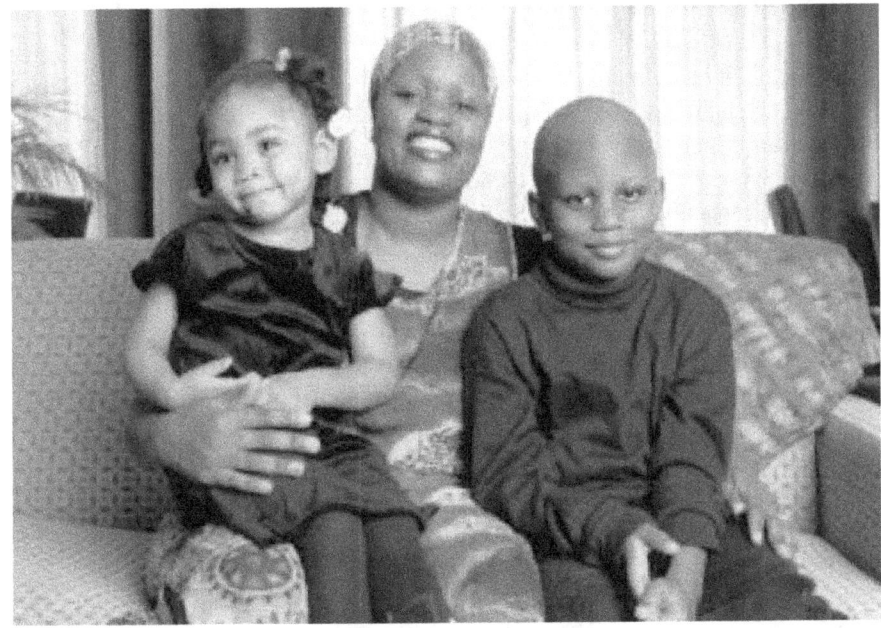

"Quitting is hard work. But I did it for myself and for my children. I knew that they would be proud of me for doing my best to quit."

Many state health agencies and private groups have programs to help smokers quit. There are classes in the community, and some government and private groups offer free telephone quitlines. Doctors, local hospitals, and health plans also have resources. Some are free and others are low cost.

However, not all quit-smoking programs are worth your time. Do not be fooled by programs that promise great success in quitting without any work on your part. They are probably just trying to take your money. If you have questions about a quit-smoking program, just ask your doctor or pharmacist.

Switching to a so-called "light" cigarette is not a good idea either. Studies show that "light" cigarettes have just as many harmful chemicals as regular cigarettes. There is no such thing as a safe cigarette.

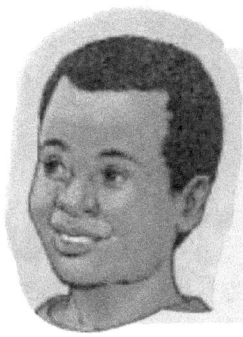

If You Want to Help

"If family members want to know more about quitting smoking, tell them you'll look up stuff on the computer. If there is no computer at home, try the library."

The First Few Days Can Be Tough

Things will get better soon. The "quitting blues" do not last forever. The pangs of giving up cigarettes tend to be strongest during the first week. You may not feel like yourself or may cough more at first. The worst part will be over soon—2 to 3 weeks after you smoke your last cigarette. After a month, you will feel better than you felt when you smoked. So, be patient. Take it one day at a time.

If You Have	What to Try
Urges to smoke	Wait it out—whether you smoke or not, the strong urge to smoke will pass in a few minutes. Remind yourself of all the reasons why you want to stop smoking. Say a prayer. Do a brief meditation. Repeat a favorite poem or verse.
Trouble paying attention	Go easy on yourself. You'll get your focus back soon enough. Break big jobs into small parts. Take a break and come back to the task a little later.
Tense, restless feelings	Take a quiet walk. Work in the garden. Listen to some soothing music. Take a shower or bath if possible. Arrange some flowers.
Frustration and anger	Get away from the problem. Exercise to blow off steam. Close your eyes and imagine something soothing and pleasant. Escape for a moment. Think about that peaceful image and nothing else.
Trouble sleeping	Try deep breathing to relax at bedtime. Drink something warm and tasty (but without caffeine!). Take a bath.
Trouble with bowels	Add some fiber to your diet—whole grain breads, cereals, fresh fruits, and vegetables. Don't forget to drink lots of water!
Hunger, especially for sweets	Drink fruit juice. Eat low-calorie sweets and fruits. Chew some sugar-free gum. Try some licorice or peppermints.

The 5 Ds Can Help You Cope

▨ **Drink Water**

Slowly sip clear water—up to 8 glasses a day. The water helps flush nicotine out of your body.

▨ **Deep Breathe**

Take 10 slow, deep breaths—in through your nose and out ever so slowly through your mouth. Deep breathing will help you feel relaxed and in control.

▨ **Do Something Else**

Focus on being busy doing something you like besides smoking. The idea is to keep from thinking about cigarettes at all.

▨ **Discuss**

Talk with a friend or family member about what's happening to you. Tell them how you are feeling. Sharing your thoughts will help a lot.

▨ **Delay**

Allow some time. Don't reach for that cigarette right away. Count to 200 and then to 250. Urges to smoke pass in about 3 to 5 minutes. ▨

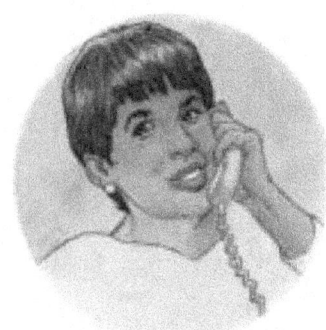

"Just called to say hi and see how you are doing."

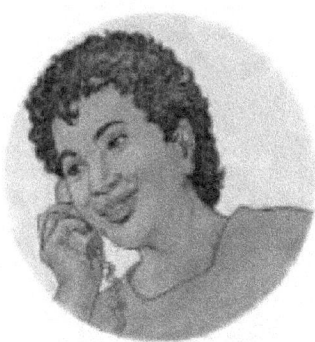

"I am hanging in there. It's hard, but I really want to make it this time."

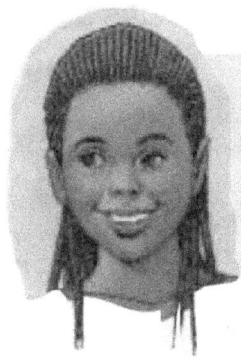

If You Want to Help

"Parents who are trying to quit smoking can be very stressed out. We kids should be on our best behavior and stay out of trouble."

25

Keeping the Weight Off

"Success doesn't come to you—you go to it."

– Marva Collins

Many people worry about gaining weight if they stop smoking. In fact, many women who don't want to get fat choose "slim" and "ultra-slim" cigarettes. Fear of gaining weight is never a good reason to keep smoking. By watching what you eat and getting more exercise, it is possible to quit smoking without gaining much or any weight at all.

You should wait until you have kicked smoking for good before starting on a diet. But it makes sense to avoid extra snacking and to do more exercise like walking.

Drinking water is necessary for good health. It is even more important for people who quit smoking. Water helps the body get rid of leftover nicotine. Try to drink at least 8 glasses of water each day, especially right after your Quit Day. Stay away from caffeinated coffee, tea, and colas.

Some People Do Gain Weight When They Stop Smoking—Here's Why...

- Your sense of taste and smell improves. Foods taste better.

- You may start to crave sweets with lots of calories.

- Your body needs 100 to 200 calories fewer a day when you quit smoking.

- You may start putting food in your mouth instead of a cigarette.

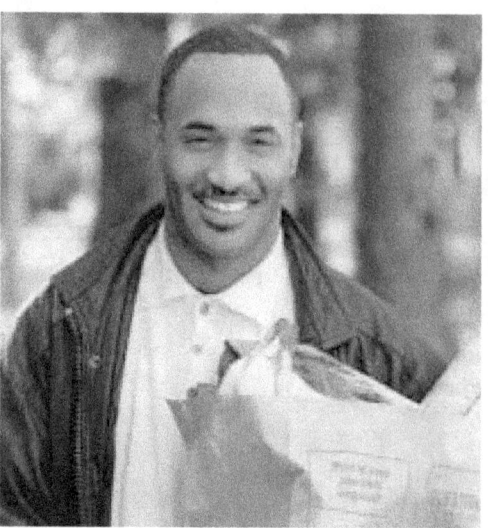

"After I quit smoking, I watched what I ate. Mostly, I tried to cut back on fatty and fried foods. I only gained 3 or 4 pounds. It really didn't bother me."

Watching What You Eat Is Only Half of It— The Other Half Is Exercise

Keeping extra pounds off is easier if you exercise. Staying active also helps you quit smoking.

Exercise does not have to be a big deal. Just do more than you were doing before. Walking is always a good idea. It gives you the chance to be alone—or to be with someone. It gives you time to think things over or to think about nothing at all. All you need are good walking shoes and a place to walk where you feel safe.

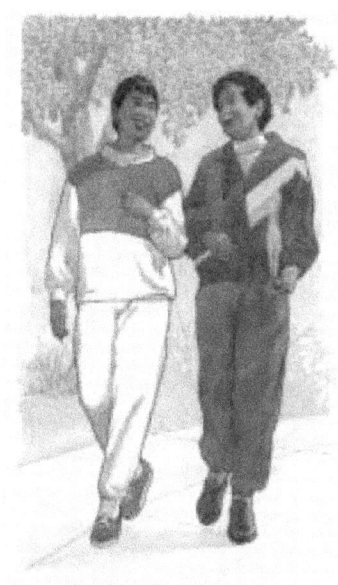

Walking with a friend is fun and a good way to stay in shape.

Here Are Some Ways to Cut Down on Calories

- Broil or bake foods when possible.
- Drain extra fat from foods that are fried.
- Cut excess fat from meat before cooking.
- Ask for sauces, gravies, and salad dressings "on the side."
- Go easy on biscuits, rolls, and breads.
- Boil or steam vegetables, and eat lots of them.
- Try not to use margarine or butter.
- Avoid meals that are full of sugars and starches.
- Switch to sherbet or frozen yogurt instead of ice cream.
- Use mustard in place of mayonnaise or sandwich spread.
- Buy tuna packed in water, not oil.

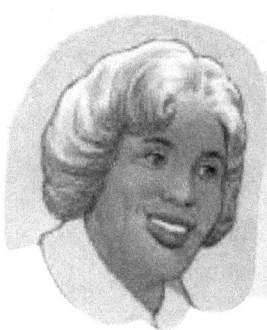

If You Want to Help
"Don't go on a cake and pie baking spree when someone is trying to quit smoking."

How to Stay Quit When You Want to Smoke

"If there is no struggle, there is no progress."

– Frederick Douglass

It takes time to get over the urge to smoke. The urges will be strongest in the places where you smoked the most. In the beginning, you may want to avoid places where you used to smoke. After a while, the urges will get a lot weaker.

Avoid smoking even one cigarette. While a single cigarette may not doom your efforts to quit, any smoking makes it easier to backslide into addiction. It is not worth the risk.

If you do get the urge to smoke, don't act on it. Instead, write down what you will do instead of smoking. It may be as simple as reaching for a toothpick instead of a cigarette. You could say a prayer or go outside for a short walk.

Some people who are still smoking may try to get you smoking again. Be ready to keep saying **NO**. Your life and your health are at stake. And no matter how much you miss your cigarettes, don't start smoking cigars or "light" cigarettes. And don't start using spit tobacco. All tobacco is bad.

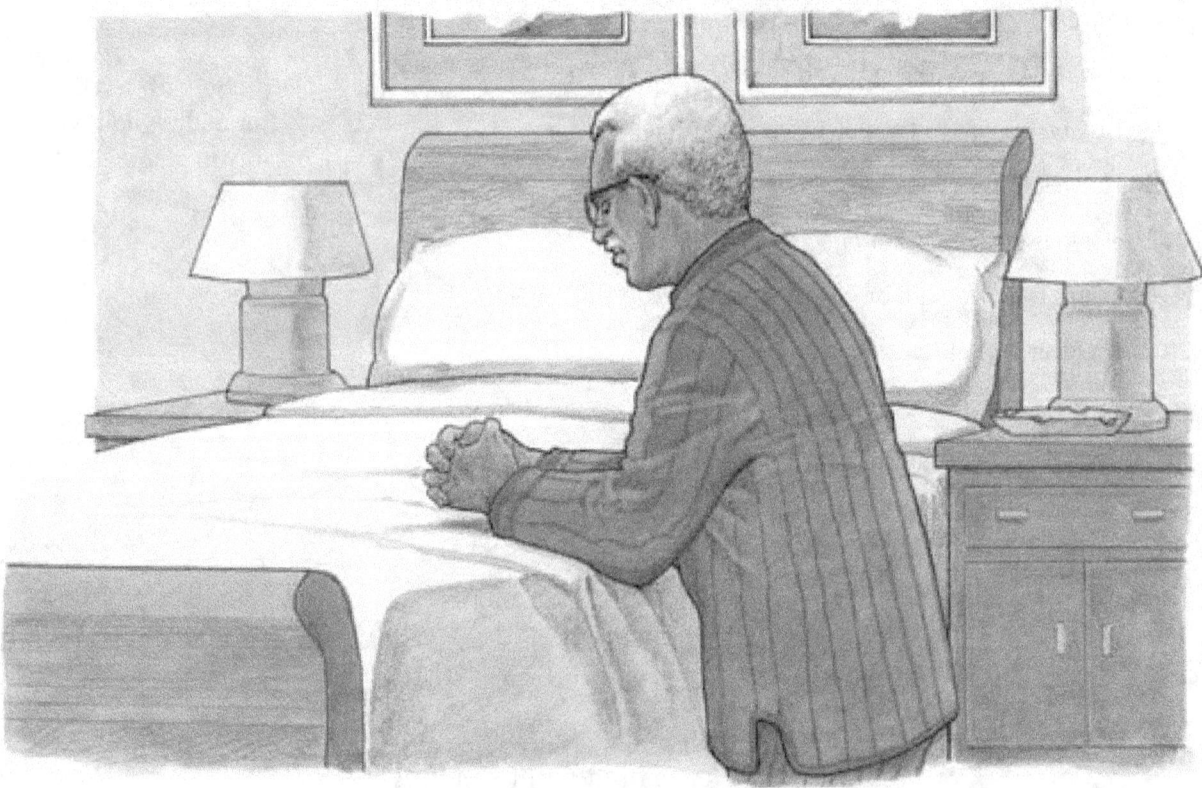

Praying helps some people meet difficult challenges, like ending addiction to tobacco.

Making It to 2 Weeks

If you have stopped smoking for 2 weeks, congratulations! You have made it through the hardest part. To stay smoke-free, stick to what got you this far. By now you should be enjoying some of the good things that come from quitting. You may already have noticed that you are coughing less and have more lung power. You should have more energy and a new sense of freedom and pride.

If you have been taking medication to help you quit, continue for at least 6 to 8 weeks—that's the time needed for the medicine to help you stay tobacco-free.

What if you slip? Try not to—not even once. But if you do smoke a cigarette or two, catch yourself and get right back on track. Don't let guilt lead you back to regular smoking. Be patient with yourself. One or more slips do not mean failure.

- Think about why you slipped and how to avoid it next time.
- Get rid of any leftover cigarettes.
- Try to spend time away from people who are still smoking.
- Call a quitline for help.

Just don't give up. Quitting takes practice. Smoking is tough to beat. Many people do not quit for good on the first try, but each try is another step toward success. You can quit. Hundreds of thousands of African American men and women already have.

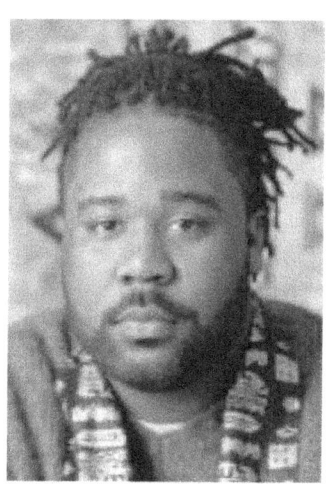

"I did OK until I was laid off. I felt like I needed my old crutch—cigarettes. Then I remembered how far I'd come. I made up my mind to stay quit."

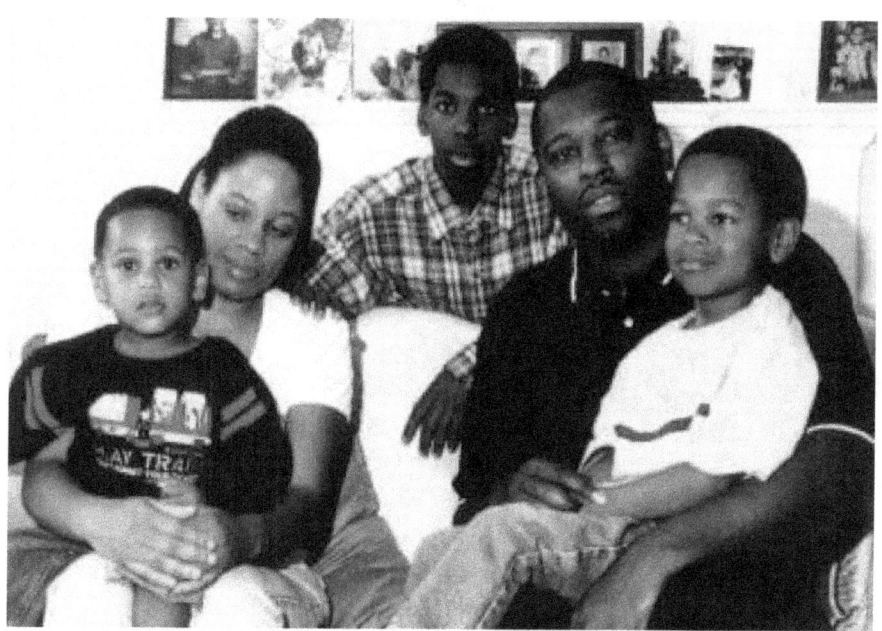

"No question about it—we wanted to give up trying. We thought about our family. We prayed about it. In 2 weeks, we felt fine."

If You Start Smoking Again

Black people quit smoking every day. But not everyone stays quit. Some return to smoking. In fact, African Americans have a harder time staying quit than other groups. No one knows why. It may simply be the stresses of everyday life...like keeping a job, juggling family demands, and dealing with race discrimination.

The medical term for going back to an addictive behavior is "relapse." It is similar for all kinds of addictive drugs—from cocaine to cigarettes. For some people, going back to smoking happens because they just can't get over wanting a cigarette. Often that happens in the first 2 weeks. For others, going back to smoking can happen months or even years after they have quit.

How Your Body Changes When You Quit Smoking	
Within 20 minutes:	• Blood pressure and pulse rate decrease • Body temperature of hands and feet increases
Within 24 to 48 hours:	• Chance of a heart attack decreases • Ability to smell and taste improves
Within 2 weeks to 3 months:	• Circulation improves • Walking becomes easier
Within 1 to 9 months:	• Coughing decreases in most people • Sinus congestion, fatigue, and shortness of breath decrease
Within 1 year:	• Added risk of heart disease drops by half
Within 5 to 15 years:	• Risk of stroke drops to that of people who have never smoked
Within 10 years:	• The risk of cancer of the lung, mouth, throat, esophagus, bladder, kidney, and pancreas also decreases
Within 15 years:	• Risk of coronary heart disease is now similar to that of people who have never smoked • Risk of death returns to nearly the level of people who have never smoked

Learn to Deal With Stress

When a former smoker goes back to smoking, it is often because of a stressful event. That is why it is so important to learn how to manage stress as a part of quitting smoking and staying quit. When life takes a turn for the worse, smoking a cigarette may seem to relieve the stress. The truth is that smoking actually keeps the body in a stressed state and causes more problems than it solves. Deep breathing and exercise are much better ways to reduce stress than cigarettes.

"I started smoking again right after my accident. But I didn't let that slip defeat me. I quit again. I haven't smoked for 10 years."

Stress isn't the only reason why people return to smoking after being quit. Happiness, boredom, loneliness, and even being around people who are smoking and drinking at a party can trigger a return to cigarettes.

What to Do

If you have been quit for a while but find yourself smoking again, act quickly:

- If you have smoked only a few cigarettes, quit again right away.

- If you are smoking at your old level, set a new Quit Day within a month or so.

- Think about what worked before, and try to figure out what you could do better.

- Ask your doctor or pharmacist if there are any other products to help smokers quit.

- Talk with a pastor or counselor.

- Read *Pathways to Freedom* again to see if there is anything you missed.

Remember, if you quit once, then you can quit again—but for good this time.

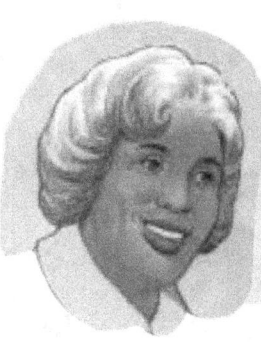

If You Want to Help

"An ex-smoker who starts smoking again needs encouragement to try again—not your criticism."

Community Organization

We Must Teach, Organize, and Take Action!

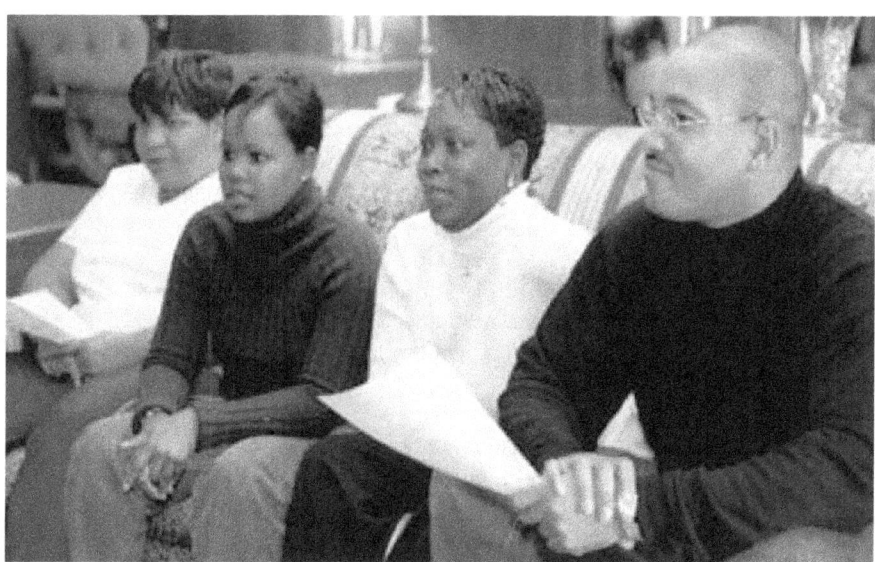

"Educating the community about the dangers of tobacco is as easy as talking to your neighbors and friends."

"Harambee" is a Swahili word from Africa that means "We must pull together." That is what we have to do to solve the tobacco problem.

Most African Americans do not smoke. Yet all of us are affected in some way by tobacco. Tobacco is part of our history. It was a major crop in the South during slavery. Tobacco companies hired Black people in good jobs. Over the years, many African Americans have worked for tobacco companies or on tobacco farms. Tobacco paid our bills.

For decades, we accepted the tobacco companies. These companies gave hundreds of thousands of dollars to Black cultural and educational programs. We really thought the tobacco companies were our friends. We did not realize their products caused disease and death.

Fighting the Tobacco Companies Is Not Easy

It is hard to fight an industry that gives us money and jobs—because the Black community needs money and jobs. But times are changing.

We can break the hold that tobacco has on our loved ones and on our community. Following are some strategies that have worked.

Fighting Back and Winning

"No matter how long the night, the day is sure to come."

– Congolese proverb

All around the nation, Black people are fighting back against the companies that sell cigarettes—and winning.

The first major victory was in 1990 with Uptown cigarettes. Uptown was a high-tar, menthol cigarette brand advertised for African Americans. It was going to be sold in Philadelphia. But the Black community fought back. As a result, not a single Uptown cigarette was ever sold in Philadelphia, or anywhere else.

Success happened in other cities. In Boston, Chicago, Los Angeles, and Atlanta, new menthol cigarettes for Blacks were introduced. They had names like X cigarettes and Camel Menthols. The people fought back against those brands, too.

Black people held sit-ins to protest cigarette ads. They took part in letter-writing campaigns against new menthol brands. Black churches held Smoke-free Sabbaths. They asked people to make their homes smoke-free. There were church services to remember loved ones who had died from tobacco. Some pastors and community leaders even whitewashed tobacco billboards.

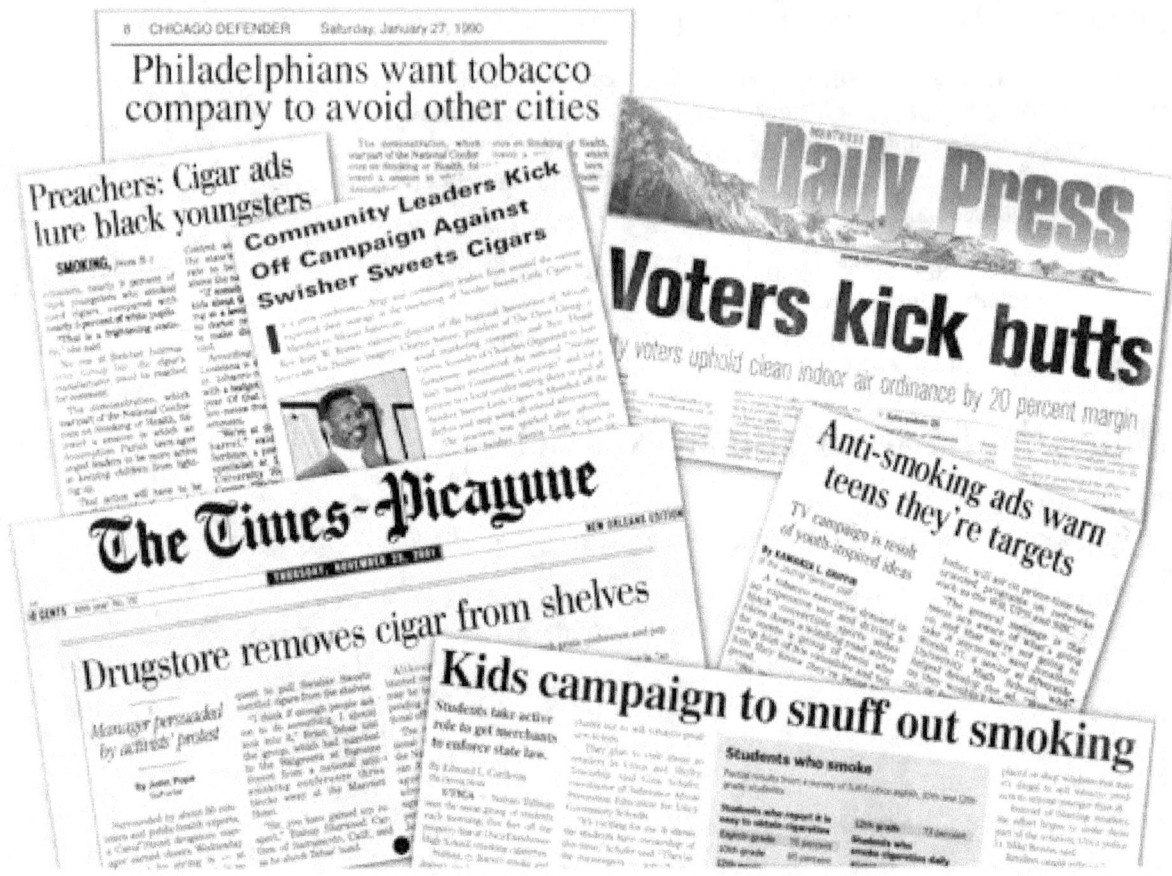

Communities Organized and Became More Powerful

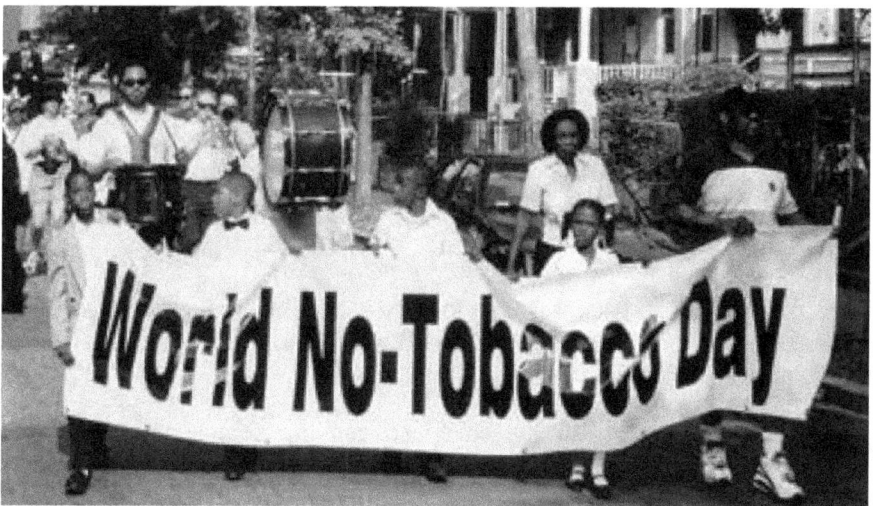

Organizing to promote a tobacco-free world.

- Black pastors preached from their pulpits about the dangers of tobacco.

- Black leaders said **NO** to money from tobacco companies.

- Black parents joined in protest marches against new cigarette brands and cigarette ads.

- Black children made their own ads about the lies tobacco companies tell.

Black people said **NO** to the tobacco companies. With each success, Black communities got stronger and healthier.

"Health is a more active concern among Blacks than Whites.... Fortunately, for this industry, this health concern does not translate strongly to anti-smoking attitudes...."

− *R. J. Reynolds Tobacco Company*

The Power to Make a Difference

"The need for change bulldozed a road down the center of my mind."
— *Maya Angelou*

In our communities, smoking is just one of the problems we face every day. We worry about many things—lack of jobs, poor housing, schools that don't teach our children, racism, drugs, and crime. All these problems need our time and energy.

But fighting against tobacco is something we can do right now. Why? Because smoking is a problem we can solve. Because smoking kills more of our people than anything else.

We can end deaths and diseases from tobacco if we all work together. Then, we can use these skills to fight other problems that our community faces. As our people become healthier, we can do great things.

Here are some ways that you and your friends can join the fight against tobacco. No one expects you to do everything on the list. Just pick one or two things to start. ▮▮

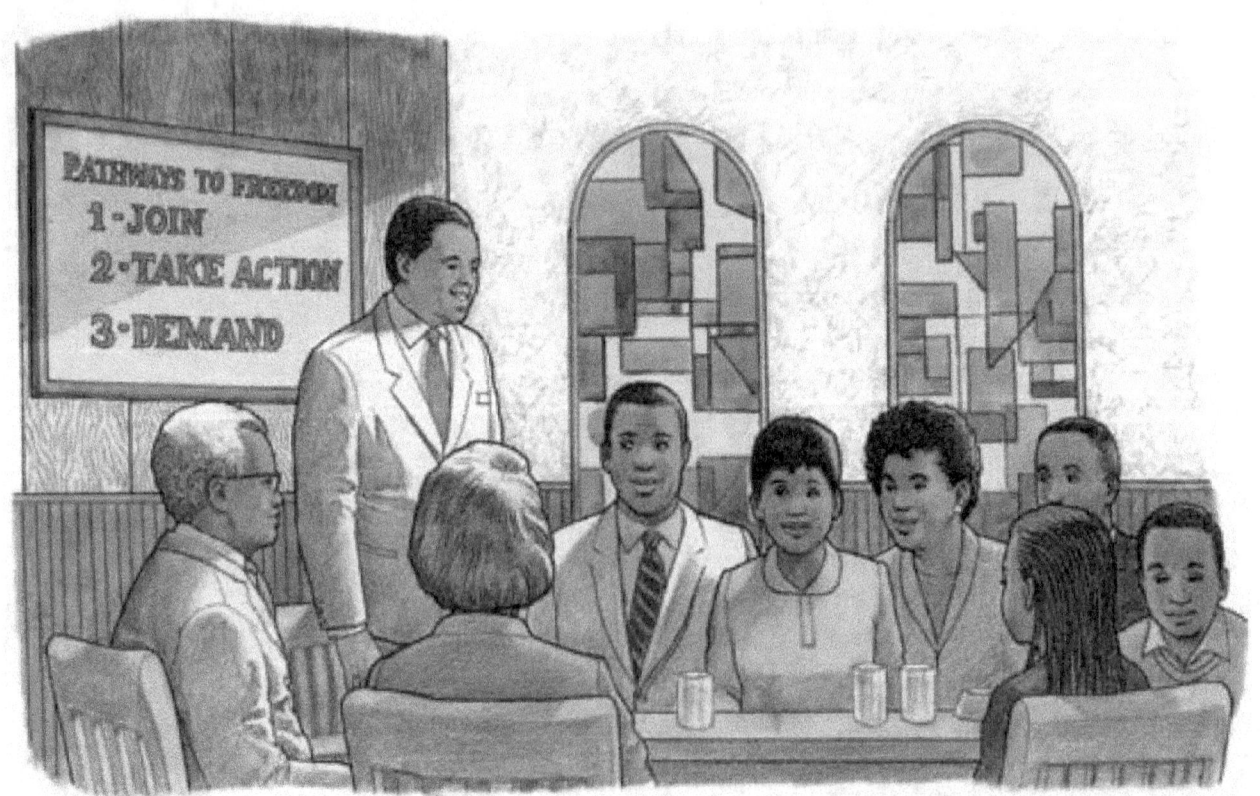

Places of worship and community centers are places where people can come together to make their neighborhoods stronger and healthier.

Things We Can Do to Help

1 **JOIN** with others to stop the sale of cigarettes to children and teenagers in stores and through vending machines. In every state, selling cigarettes to anyone under 18 is against the law.

2 **MEET** with store owners and ask them to remove tobacco ads that young people can see.

3 **MAKE SURE** schools teach the dangers of using tobacco. Our children need the facts so they can live healthy and tobacco-free lives.

4 **HOLD** programs for churches and mosques, fraternities and sororities, civic leagues, clubs, and community groups on the dangers of tobacco and what communities can do.

5 **WORK** with union leaders and company bosses to have smoke-free rules and quit-smoking programs on the job. Get health plans to cover quit-smoking medicines and classes.

6 **ASK** health clinics, doctors, and local hospitals to hold low-cost or free clinics for people who want to quit smoking.

7 **HELP** groups in the community say no to "gifts" from tobacco companies. Look for other ways to get money for youth programs, reading tutors, scholarships, and other things the community needs.

8 **SUPPORT** efforts to increase taxes on tobacco. Make sure that money is spent in Black communities to end smoking and to help the community in other ways.

9 **URGE** elected officials to pass strong laws to protect communities from the dangers of secondhand smoke and support state telephone quitlines.

10 **SHARE** copies of the *Pathways to Freedom* guide. Give them to friends, neighbors, and family members.

Following the Pathways to Freedom

"Freedom is
never given,
it is won."

– A. Philip Randolph

At the beginning of this guide, three members of our family were smokers—Granddaddy, Sam, and Noreen.

Our children—Nia, M.J., and Tyrone—were all at risk for illnesses from secondhand smoke. They also were in danger of becoming smokers themselves because adults around them smoked. That has all changed.

With love and support, the smokers in our family kicked their addiction to cigarettes. Our entire family also joined with others to help make our community as tobacco-free as possible. We helped pass clean indoor air laws and higher tobacco taxes... which give us healthy air and keep more children from starting to smoke.

You and your family can do the same thing. Whoever you are, wherever you live, there is a way for you to join the fight against tobacco.

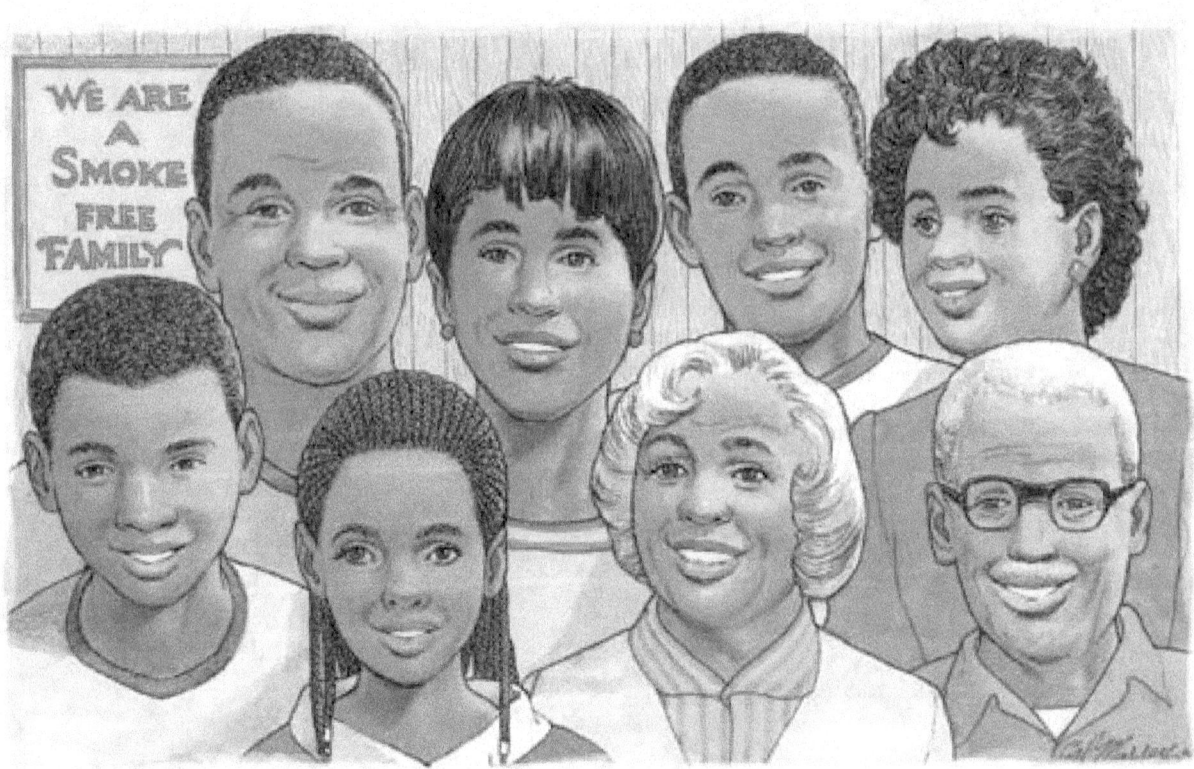

One year later, everyone in the Freeman family is healthier, happier, and smoke-free.

Respect Your Community, Keep It Tobacco-Free

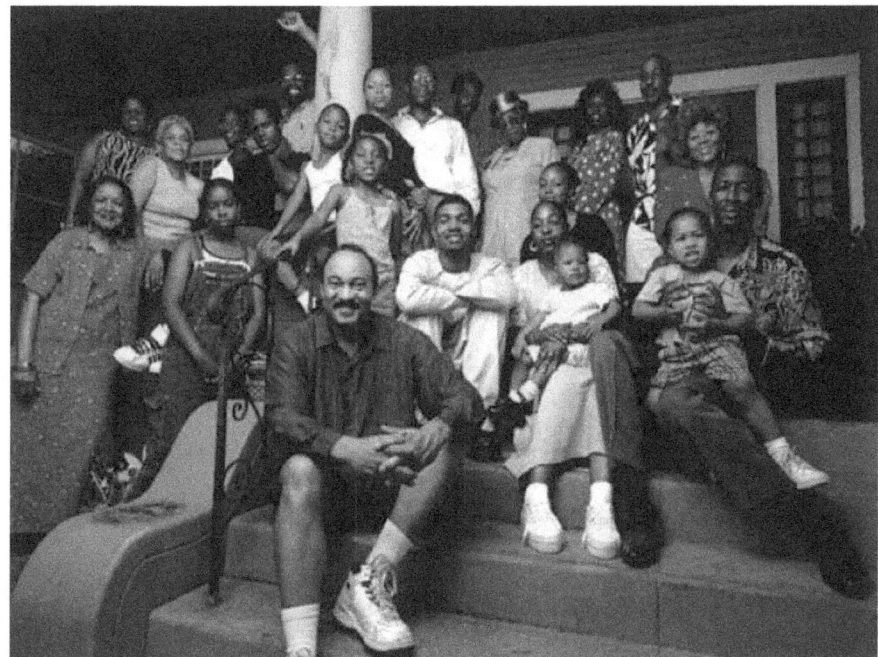

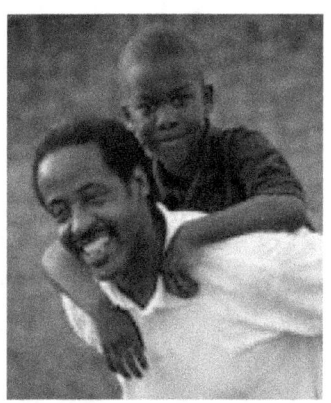

"I decided to get involved for him. We need strong healthy communities for our children."

There are many paths that each of us can take to a smoke-free future.

If you are a smoker, quit as soon as possible. Check with your state or city health department about whether your state has a free telephone quitline or other programs. Ask your doctor or a local health center if medicine and counseling are available.

If you don't smoke, help someone who is trying to quit. A survey of smokers in 2001 showed that more than 3 out of every 4 smokers in the Black community want to quit. Let's help them succeed.

Whether you are a smoker or not, get involved. There is a lot to do. Join a tobacco control group that needs your help. Get your club or neighborhood group to take a stand against tobacco in the Black community. By pulling together, we can build a healthier community where people don't have to die years before their time because of cigarettes. ▪

Help Yourself and Others Quit Smoking

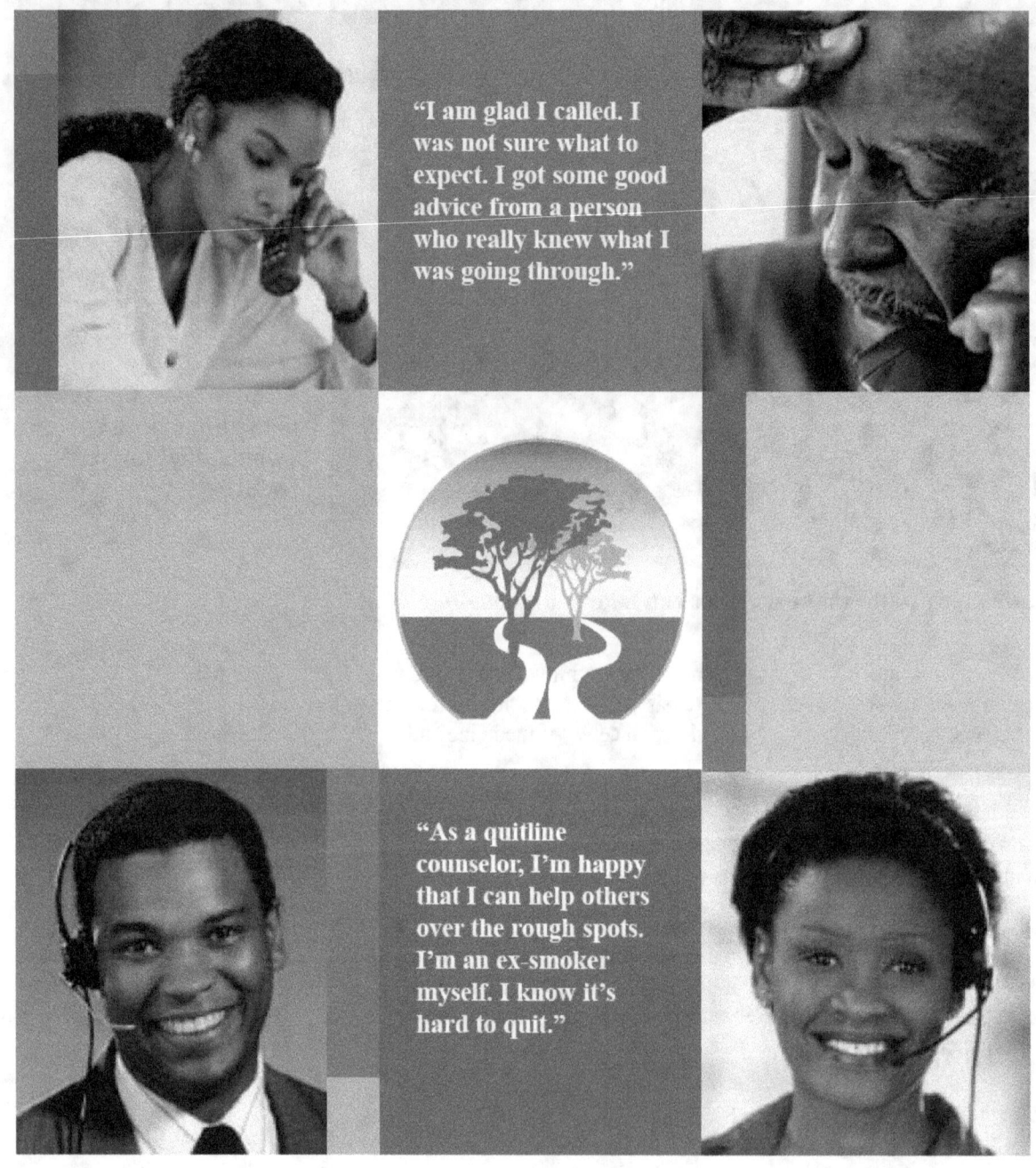

"I am glad I called. I was not sure what to expect. I got some good advice from a person who really knew what I was going through."

"As a quitline counselor, I'm happy that I can help others over the rough spots. I'm an ex-smoker myself. I know it's hard to quit."

Here Are Some Resources to Help You Quit

Call Toll-Free Numbers...

American Cancer Society
1-800-227-2345
http://www.cancer.org

National Cancer Institute
1-877-448-7848
http://www.smokefree.gov

Or Visit These Web Sites

Agency for Healthcare
Research and Quality (AHRQ)
http://www.ahrq.gov

Centers for Disease Control and
Prevention (CDC)
http://www.cdc.gov/tobacco

American Lung Association
Freedom From Smoking Online
http://www.ffsonline.org

American Legacy Foundation
http://www.americanlegacy.org

American Heart Association
http://www.americanheart.org

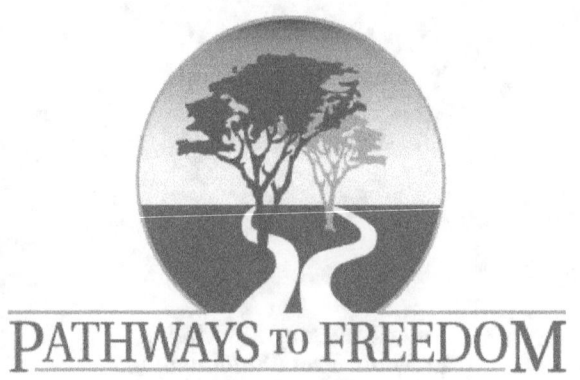

PATHWAYS TO FREEDOM

Acknowledgments

We are especially indebted to members of the *Pathways to Freedom* Advisory Committee. **First Edition:** James Barnes, Jr., Rita Butler, Russell Fletcher, Jr., Sister Patricia Haley, Vivian Hughes, Ulysses Jones, Howard T. Mallard, Jr., Ruby J. Ruffin, Regina Sidney, Wallace Stevenson, Jr., and Lillian Trump. **Second Edition:** Bishop S.C. Carthen, Sandra Headen, Denise A. James, Yvonne Lewis, Jeanne Robinson, Sylvia Rosas, Abby C. Rosenthal, Peggy Toy, and Janice R. Love.

In addition we would like to thank David Graham, Dr. Gary King, Dr. Sharon Marable, and Dr. Valerie Yerger for consultation on this publication; Cal Massey for his illustrations; and Eloisa Montes for her management and coordination of this initiative.

CREDITS

Page 7: The first two lung photographs were provided by the Medical Examiner's Office, City of Philadelphia The third lung photograph was provided by Stephen M Keller, M D , Fox Chase Cancer Center Note: The lungs are not shown true to scale; Data source: Centers for Disease Control and Prevention Smoking-attributable Mortality, Morbidity, and Economic Costs (SAMMEC): Adult SAMMEC software, 2002 Available at http://www cdc gov/tobacco/sammec htm; Hyert DL, et al Deaths: Final Data for 1999 National Vital Statistics Report; Vol 49 No 8 Hyattsville, Maryland: National Center for Health Statistics 2001; Anderson, RN Deaths: Leading Causes for 1999 National Vital Statistics Reports; Vol 49 No 11 Hyattsville, Maryland: National Center for Health Statistics, 2001

Page 9: Ashtray lungs photo courtesy of Minnesota Partnership for Action Against Tobacco

Page 10: Quote Source: Brown and Williamson Tobacco Corporation (1984) Bateman M , Total Minority Marketing Plan Bates Number: 531000141-0144 Retrieved on February 28, 2002 from: http://legacy library ucsf edu/tid/eph40f00

Page 29: Family photo courtesy of South Carolina African American Tobacco Control Network

Page 35: Photograph courtesy of National Association of African Americans for Positive Imagery

Quote Source: R J Reynolds Tobacco Company (1985) Black Opportunity Analysis Bates Number: 505368425-505368482 Retrieved on January 14, 2002, from http//tobaccodocuments org/rjr/505368425-8482 html

Additional photography services were provided by Randy Santos, Randolph Photography

Cartoon concept created by Charyn Sutton; illustrated by Jay Scruggs, Comics Collaborative